PRESCRIPTION
DRUG ABUSE

Recent Titles in Health and Medical Issues Today

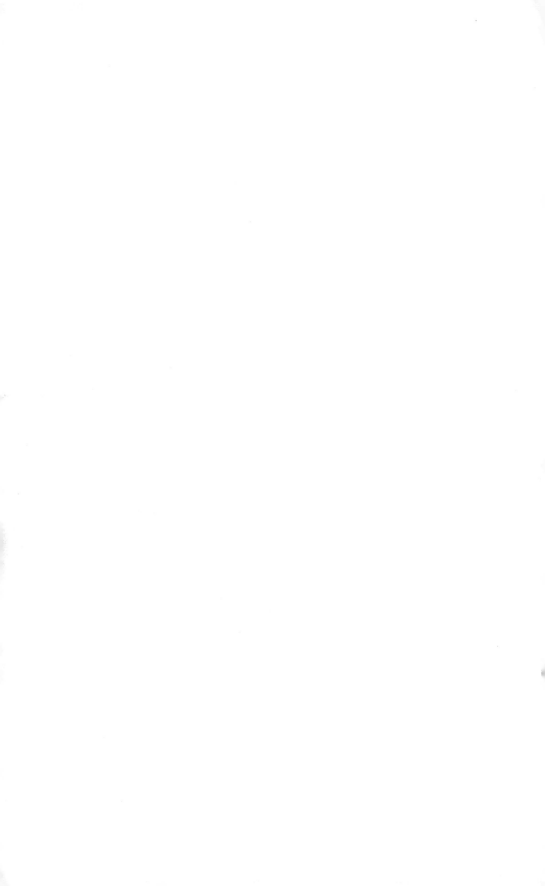

Prescription
Drug Abuse

Robert L. Bryant and Howard L. Forman

Health and Medical Issues Today

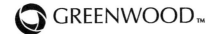 GREENWOOD™

An Imprint of ABC-CLIO, LLC

Santa Barbara, California • Denver, Colorado

Library of Congress Cataloging-in-Publication Data

Names: Bryant, Robert L. (Robert Leslie), 1982- author. | Forman, Howard
   L., author.
Title: Prescription drug abuse / Robert L. Bryant and Howard L. Forman.
Description: Santa Barbara, California : Greenwood, an imprint of ABC-CLIO,
   LLC, [2019] | Series: Health and medical issues today | Includes
   bibliographical references and index.
Identifiers: LCCN 2019025684 (print) | LCCN 2019025685 (ebook) | ISBN
   9781440859199 | ISBN 9781440859205 (ebook)
Subjects: LCSH: Medication abuse.
Classification: LCC RM146.5 .B78 2019 (print) | LCC RM146.5 (ebook) | DDC
   362.29/9—dc23
LC record available at https://lccn.loc.gov/2019025684
LC ebook record available at https://lccn.loc.gov/2019025685

ISBN: 978–1–4408–5919–9 (print)
        978–1–4408–5920–5 (ebook)

23 22 21 20 19   1 2 3 4 5

This book is also available as an eBook.

Greenwood
An Imprint of ABC-CLIO, LLC

ABC-CLIO, LLC
147 Castilian Drive
Santa Barbara, California 93117
www.abc-clio.com

This book is printed on acid-free paper ∞

Manufactured in the United States of America

This book discusses treatments (including types of medication and mental health therapies), diagnostic tests for various symptoms and mental health disorders, and organizations. The authors have made every effort to present accurate and up-to-date information. However, the information in this book is not intended to recommend or endorse particular treatments or organizations, or substitute for the care or medical advice of a qualified health professional, or used to alter any medical therapy without a medical doctor's advice. Specific situations may require specific therapeutic approaches not included in this book. For those reasons, we recommend that readers follow the advice of qualified health care professionals directly involved in their care. Readers who suspect they may have specific medical problems should consult a physician about any suggestions made in this book.

This book is dedicated to my family, friends, and mentors who supported, advised, and encouraged me throughout this writing process.
—Robert L. Bryant

In memory of my father, Arthur J. Forman MD. In honor of my mother, Susan Forman, and my wife, Shira Forman.
—Howard L. Forman

Contents

SERIES FOREWORD

Every day, the public is bombarded with information on developments in medicine and health care. Whether it is on the latest techniques in treatment or research, or on concerns over public health threats, this information directly affects the lives of people more than almost any other issue. Although there are many sources for understanding these topics—from websites and blogs to newspapers and magazines—students and ordinary citizens often need one resource that makes sense of the complex health and medical issues affecting their daily lives.

The *Health and Medical Issues Today* series provides just such a one-stop resource for obtaining a solid overview of the most controversial areas of health care in the twenty-first century. Each volume addresses one topic and provides a balanced summary of what is known. These volumes provide an excellent first step for students and laypeople interested in understanding how health care works in our society today.

Each volume is broken into several parts to provide readers and researchers with easy access to the information they need:

- Part I provides overview chapters on background information—including chapters on such areas as the historical, scientific, medical, social, and legal issues involved—that a citizen needs to intelligently understand the topic.
- Part II provides capsule examinations of the most heated contemporary issues and debates, and analyzes in a balanced manner the viewpoints held by various advocates in the debates.
- Part III provides case studies that show examples of the concepts discussed in the previous parts.

A selection of reference material, such as a timeline of important events, a directory of organizations, and a bibliography, serve as the best next step in learning about the topic at hand.

The *Health and Medical Issues Today* series strives to provide readers with all the information needed to begin making sense of some of the most important debates going on in the world today. The series includes volumes on such topics as stem-cell research, obesity, gene therapy, alternative medicine, organ transplantation, mental health, and more.

PREFACE

With the rate of prescription drug overdose deaths having increased greatly in recent years, there has been an increased demand by the general public to understand why this form of drug abuse is happening and how society can work toward better solutions. The appropriate way to address drug abuse, addiction, and intoxication has been debated for centuries, and indeed these are subjects of such societal importance that they have been addressed by the sacred texts of all major religions. Depending on the societal context, use of intoxicating substances can be viewed as a criminal act, a sacred ritual, a medical treatment, or one of many other social functions. When illegal street drugs are seen as the primary issue in drug abuse, it is easy to view drug abuse as simply a criminal activity. However, when prescription drugs recommended to patients by medical doctors increasingly become the most popular drugs of abuse, the question of how we as a society address drug abuse becomes much more complicated than a simple "Just Say No." This book serves as an entry point into the discussion of drug abuse in general as well as prescription drug abuse specifically.

This book is divided into three main sections. Part I is the Overview section, which contains five chapters that provide general knowledge about prescription drug abuse. Chapter 1 presents a broad overview of the topic, defines the different types of substance abuse, describes how prescription drug abuse differs from other forms of substance abuse, and describes the different patterns of prescription drug abuse among different populations in the United States. Chapter 2 presents a scientific explanation of how drug abuse and addiction occur, in order to describe the way in which addiction can be viewed as a disease. The next three chapters discuss specific classes of prescription drugs that are commonly abused.

Chapter 3 discusses "downer" drugs mostly in the drug class known as "sedative-hypnotics," which include drugs such as Xanax and Klonopin. Chapter 4 discusses painkillers including opioid drugs such as oxycodone and fentanyl. Chapter 5 discusses "upper" drugs and performance enhancers coming mostly from the stimulant drug class, including drugs such as Adderall and Ritalin.

Part II is the Controversy section, which goes beyond the general knowledge gained from the first section of the book and presents current controversies related to the subject of prescription drug abuse. Chapter 6 discusses the business of medicine, describing how corporate interests and financial dealings within the medical and pharmaceutical industries have influenced rates of prescription drug abuse. Chapter 7 discusses the treatment philosophies of prescription drug abuse and compares harm reduction strategies to abstinence strategies. Chapter 8 discusses the War on Drugs and government policies that have attempted to address prescription drug abuse. Chapter 9 presents three cases of prescription drug abuse adapted from the stories of real patients in order to illustrate the complex problems of prescription drug abuse at the level of individual people.

Part III features case studies that support the reader's understanding of the first two sections. Following this section are a glossary of terms used in this book, suggested readings for those who wish to further their knowledge, a timeline of important events in the history of prescription drug abuse, and an index to help readers locate specific topics in the text.

* * *

This book was written by two psychiatrists working at a large, academic hospital system in the Bronx, New York. As a result, our understanding of addiction and mental illness has been shaped by the stories of the patients we treat in this diverse, dense borough. Even for professionals, it can be easy among the statistics about the drugs and addiction to think of substance abuse in the abstract. One can easily lose sight of the real, living people who are behind the numbers. Likewise, headlines and stories people tell each other about "junkies" and "thugs" can often paint two-dimensional pictures of people that do not capture the full complexity of how this person came to be trapped in a vicious cycle of drug use. However, working as psychiatrists has afforded us the opportunity to discuss the difficulties of drug abuse and mental illness as they are experienced firsthand by our patients. Some patients struggle with addiction themselves, and they speak with us about the difficulty this brings to their lives. Other patients are the loved ones of people with substance abuse problems, and so they describe the ways their lives are affected by the drug use of others. These patient interactions have informed every aspect of the writing of this text, and it is our hope to convey with this writing that beyond the headlines and pages of government statistics, there are always human beings. Every person has experienced a childhood. Every person has experienced love, hate, fear, and pain. Every person has a network of friends, family, coworkers, or other people that have been affected in one way or another by the drug use. No matter what race, religion, or social class that someone belongs to, whether or not someone has used drugs themselves, every person is exposed to the problems caused by drug abuse at some point in their lives. By use of perspectives gained from our clinical practice as well as by inclusion of cultural references, we hope this book illuminates the human side of prescription drug abuse at the same time as it explains the science behind it.

Robert L. Bryant, MD
Howard L. Forman, MD

PART I

Overview

CHAPTER 1

The Prescribed Epidemic: An Overview of Prescription Drug Abuse

One of the principal concerns of public health officials across the world is to identify and to combat the spread of epidemics, which are outbreaks of disease that spread rapidly among numerous people in a short amount of time and result in large populations of people with the disease. For example, in late 2014, the world saw the beginnings of what would be known as the West African Ebola outbreak, and the dreaded *Ebolavirus* began spreading exponentially to many populations in West Africa (particularly in Sierra Leone, Liberia, and Guinea). Fears that an Ebola epidemic might spread to the United States reached a fever pitch in the news media as well as in the conversations of average Americans. Ebola can spread quickly, it can kill quickly, and its effects on humans are often gruesome. Days to weeks after contracting the virus, people begin to have flulike symptoms of fever, malaise, fatigue, muscle ache, headache, and sore throat. This can then proceed to onset of diarrhea, vomiting, a rash consisting of little red bumps. Finally, in the worst cases, the blood loses the ability to coagulate, which can result in large bruises, bloody vomit, bloody diarrhea, and even bleeding into the whites of the eyes. Between March 2014 and April 2016, by which time the outbreak was effectively contained, 11,325 deaths from Ebola occurred in West Africa, mostly in the countries of Sierra Leone, Liberia, and Guinea.

The total death toll from the Ebola outbreak was tragically high, and if it were not for the heroic efforts by physicians and policy makers in the global health system to contain the virus and eradicate it, surely many more would have died. Through these preventive measures, spread of the epidemic to the United States was largely evaded. During that epidemic, there were a total of four confirmed cases of Ebola in the United States.

One of those four people died from the disease, and the other three recovered and survived.

During the same time period as the Ebola outbreak, while the attention of the news media was so highly focused on concerns that the virus might reach North America, another less publicized epidemic was smoldering quietly in the back rooms of American households, mostly out of public view and off the front pages of the newspapers. This quieter epidemic, only then just starting to break into the awareness of the average American, became apparent when officials started to notice a very sharp rise in the number of overdose deaths caused by taking too large a dose of opioid drugs. According to the Centers for Disease Control and Prevention (CDC), in 2014 alone, there were reportedly 28,646 overdose deaths involving opioid drugs in the United States. This phenomenon became what is now commonly called the opioid epidemic or the opioid crisis.

To place the severity of the opioid epidemic in context, this means that in one year, 2014, there were over 17,000 more deaths in the United States caused by opioid drug overdose than the total number of all the deaths that occurred during the entire two-year Ebola outbreak in West Africa. While awareness of the American opioid epidemic continues to grow, sadly so does the death toll. In 2016, the number of deaths in the United States due to opioid overdose rose even higher to a staggering 42,249.

The opioid epidemic plays out in cities and towns all across the country. Economically depressed rural areas and small towns have been some of the hardest hit. In Huntington, West Virginia, a small town of about 50,000 residents in the heart of Appalachia, there have been on average two to three drug overdose deaths per day in recent years, largely caused by drugs in the opioid drug class. On one particularly bad day in 2016, officials found 26 people dead from opioid overdose. It has been estimated that about 1 in 10 residents there misuses opioids.

What has been notable and surprising to many about this epidemic is that most of the rise in drug overdose deaths starting from the early 2000s was caused by an increase of overdoses of prescription opioid medications, not the street drugs that are commonly associated with overdosing and drug abuse in popular culture. The term "opioid" refers to a class of pain-relieving drugs that includes prescription medications such as oxycodone, the active ingredient in various brand-name drugs including Percocet and OxyContin. In the world of illegal street drugs, another opioid drug is also sold that contributes to the deaths in the opioid epidemic as well: heroin. What may surprise many readers is that the overdose deaths involving heroin have been far outpaced by the number of drug overdose deaths involving prescription opioid pain medications for nearly two decades. How did legal prescription pain medications end up leading to so many more deaths than an illegal drug as vilified as heroin?

THE DRUG OVERDOSE EPIDEMIC AND THE COMPLEX ROLE OF PRESCRIPTION DRUGS

Unfortunately, the epidemic of opioid overdose is but one part of a greater drug overdose epidemic this country is currently facing. The total number of drug overdose deaths in the United States in 2017 rose to around 72,000. This means that number has quadrupled since the year 2000, when the yearly total was around 17,415. According to the Drug Enforcement Agency, every day, 129 people die from drug overdose in the United States. Far more people now die from drug overdose deaths than die from car collisions, as there were 35,485 people who died from motor vehicle accidents in 2015. Deaths from drug overdose also far eclipse the total number of homicides in the United States, of which there were 15,696 in 2016.

The total number of drug overdose deaths for 2017 reported above includes overdoses from street drugs as well as prescription medications; and contrary to popular belief, it is the rise in abuse of prescription drugs that is responsible for much of the recent rise in drug overdose deaths. The major drugs that result in overdose death are prescription opioids, heroin, cocaine; stimulants such as methamphetamine; and prescription benzodiazepines (a class of sedative drugs) such as Xanax. In the United States, the number of overdose deaths involving prescription opioids has surpassed the number of overdose deaths involving heroin ever since the year 2002. In fact, overdose of prescription medications is now involved in more deaths per year than heroin and cocaine combined. In 2015, there were about 13,000 drug overdose deaths involving heroin and about 6,500 involving overdose from cocaine. By comparison to the about 17,636 deaths from prescription opioid pain medications that year (excluding non-methadone synthetics such as fentanyl). An additional 9,580 deaths in 2015 involved synthetic opioids such as the pain medication fentanyl. Fentanyl, a prescription opioid dozens of times more potent than heroin, is often used for terminally ill cancer patients, and it has recently found its way into the illegal drug trade. Altogether, the total number of drug overdose deaths from opioid medications in 2015 was greater than 27,000. (Although it should be noted that fentanyl, once predominantly a prescription-only drug, has been increasingly produced illegally by secret labs in China and Mexico since 2013 and sold on the black market. Thus, what was once a prescription drug produced and sold by pharmaceutical companies is now being produced and sold illegally by criminal organizations.) Prescription benzodiazepines were involved in about 9,000 overdose deaths in 2015, a rate significantly higher than that of cocaine. In 2016, there were 7,500 overdose deaths involving psychostimulants with abuse potential, such as methamphetamine, MDMA, and prescription stimulants like methylphenidate (Ritalin) or amphetamine (Adderall).

Many of these overdose deaths were not the result of taking too much of a single drug. Rather, it is often a combination of drugs, also known as polysubstance use, that can lead to overdose, as the cumulative effects of multiple drug types add together and result in fatal effects. In these cases, it is not accurate to say one particular drug caused the overdose, and so the statistics describe that the drug was "involved in" the overdose. For example, benzodiazepines and opioids can both decrease the respiratory drive as a side effect, and so when they are both taken together, they can be particularly dangerous by causing the user to stop breathing. Mixing benzodiazepines or opioids with alcohol can also be particularly dangerous.

To complicate matters, it is becoming increasingly clear that counterfeit prescription drugs are also entering the picture to add to the drug overdose crisis. These drugs are look-alike reproductions of brand-name medications, which may or may not actually contain the same compound. Law enforcement officials in recent years have found and confiscated illegal pill presses during drug raids. For example, a dealer may offer to sell what appears to be a pill of the prescription drug OxyContin, when in actuality it may be an imitation pill consisting of pressed fentanyl with other substances. Illegally produced fentanyl is increasingly added to bags of heroin or cocaine in attempts to stretch a dealer's supply. Deaths in the United States involving illegally produced synthetic fentanyl have risen exponentially each year, from an estimated 3,105 deaths in 2013 to an estimated 29,406 in 2017.

Since 1992, the rate that addictive drugs are prescribed and the rate that prescription drugs are abused have both risen simultaneously. Prescription opioids are the most commonly abused prescription drugs, and the number of people abusing them in the United States more than doubled from 4.9 million in 1992 to 12.5 million in 2012. In 2012, there were about 259 million opioid prescriptions written, which was equal to the total number of adults in the country. There were 6 million people who reported abusing prescription sedatives such as benzodiazepines in 2012, and 3.3 million people who reported abusing stimulants such as Adderall or Ritalin. The lifetime rate of medically appropriate use of prescription stimulants is the same as the lifetime rate of abuse of prescription stimulants. For example, a report from the Drug Enforcement Agency noted that a 67% increase in nonmedical use of Adderall occurred between the years 2006 and 2011, which was correlated with an increase in ADHD diagnoses of 7.8% between the years 2003 and 2011.

From these drug overdose statistics above, it is clear that the ravages of drug abuse are increasing at an alarming rate in the United States. Perhaps what is also clear is that street drugs, those produced and sold on the black market as part of a criminal enterprise and the traditional targets of the War on Drugs—such as cocaine, marijuana, or heroin—are only a portion of the nation's drug problem. Prescription drug abuse has risen in the past three decades as an ever more dangerous and harmful phenomenon in the United States. In addition to the numerous overdose deaths listed above, the drug overdose crisis carries additional casualties for the friends and loved ones of those that died, since, for example, children may be left behind who have lost a parent. The rise of prescription drug abuse complicates the popular narrative about the nature of drug abuse and about which drugs are dangerous. It calls for new ways of thinking about the problem of drug abuse in general and how it can be addressed. Though the threat is clear, the problem is complex and its solutions are difficult.

DEFINING DRUG ABUSE

Drug abuse in general is more complex to define than one might initially think. The line between what is abuse and what is not abuse is sometimes grey because many different patterns of drug use exist, and whether or not a particular pattern of use constitutes "abuse" is sometimes a matter of perspective. Furthermore, abuse does not always mean the same as addiction. For example, irresponsible use of a drug like alprazolam (Xanax) by taking it at a party while drinking alcohol and then driving home in a car full of friends would be considered prescription drug abuse because the behavior is highly dangerous and the use of Xanax is not appropriate. However, this person does not necessarily have an addiction to Xanax because of this one instance of poor judgment. Likewise, it is not always clear-cut how to describe a person who abuses drugs. It is easy to think of people as being in either of two categories: a drug user or not a drug user. Some common terms used to describe drug users reflect this way of thinking—for example, the words "junkie," "drug addict," or simply an "addict." These negative stereotypes paint the picture of a person who is more like a nonperson, a ghost, or someone who is completely controlled by and defined by their drug use. In this characterization, an addict is a drain on society, immoral, unemployed, homeless, possibly violent, and essentially a criminal. In truth, there is a vast variety of types of people and patterns in the way they use and misuse drugs. The difficulty with characterizing people who use drugs as one-dimensional addicts is that it creates a blind spot into a large grey area of drug use that is dangerous but does not qualify as being addicted. Likewise, the level and effect of addiction can vary depending on the person and circumstances. Some addictions reach severity to where they consume a person's entire purpose in life. By contrast, a person may be physically addicted to a prescription drug in the sense that the person might have a withdrawal syndrome if he or she stopped the drug, but this does not necessarily mean this person is abusing the drug. (As a further complication, in some contexts, such as in the organizations Alcohol Anonymous and Narcotics Anonymous, the members are encouraged to identify themselves as "addicts" as a way to take ownership of their addiction. Thus, in that context, "addict" takes on a positive connotation. However, it should be noted that this only holds true among members of the organizations when they refer to themselves as addicts. Labeling oneself an addict as a way to fight addiction is empowering. Labeling another as a dehumanized "addict" is disenfranchising.)

In order to begin sorting out what is meant by prescription drug abuse, it is useful to begin by defining the term "drug" itself, which has different meanings depending on the context. Perhaps the most basic definition of a drug is that it is any chemical substance that causes a change in the function of the body but that is not food. In the strictly medical sense of the word, one could also say a drug is any substance with a medicinal purpose against disease and to increase well-being. These definitions give a sense of the word "drug" as used by the Food and Drug Administration (FDA), the regulatory agency that is responsible for ensuring that new medicines sold in the United States are proven to be safe and effective. In everyday language, "medication" is the term more often used to denote these sorts of drugs that one gets prescribed from the doctor or that one buys over the counter to treat a cold, for example. The difference between medication and all other types of drugs is that medicine is used to treat or prevent disease. Prescription drugs are drugs that in general are legally obtained only through receiving a prescription by a practitioner such as a medical doctor. These are often not dispensed directly by the practitioner, but instead are usually dispensed by a pharmacist. Whether or not a drug requires a prescription can vary somewhat by country.

When there is no context to suggest a neutral meaning, the word drug often has a more negative connotation. When Richard Nixon declared a "War on Drugs" in the 1970s, he was not referring to ibuprofen or penicillin, he was referring to drugs that have the potential to be abused. This is also the sense of the word drug used by the Drug Enforcement Administration (DEA), the federal law enforcement agency that works to investigate illegal drug trafficking, drug production, sales, and more. As was shown earlier, drug abuse, also known as drug misuse, is itself not a well-defined term, but broadly it means *the use of drugs in a way that is dangerous to oneself or to others.* As opposed to medications, drugs of abuse that are used for purposes other than to treat or prevent disease. Which drugs have a potential to be abused? In general, one thinks of psychoactive drugs. Psychoactive drugs are drugs that affect the function of the brain, which results in altered states of consciousness, changes in perception, mood changes, and behavioral changes. One way that psychoactive drugs can be dangerous is by causing intoxication. Intoxication is an alteration in the mind's function after taking a drug, and this can result in dangerous situations, such as overdosing or crashing a car, but it is time-limited in effect based on how long the drug lasts in the system, usu-ally several hours. Being in a state of intoxication such as this while driv-ing a car counts as drug abuse, because it is irresponsibly dangerous. Different psychoactive drugs result in different syndromes of intoxication. When used repeatedly over a long period of time, many psychoactive drugs can lead to addiction, which involves a chronic pattern of misuse, intoxication, and difficulty stopping (this topic is explored further in Chapter 2). One episode of intoxication alone does not imply addiction. Even though intoxication can potentially be a dangerous state of mind to one oneself or others, the feeling of getting "high" is often enjoyable for the user. For this reason, the use of drugs for nonmedical, pleasurable effects is called recreational use, and drugs used in this manner are called recreational drugs. The term "recreational drugs" can also include legal substances such as alcohol and tobacco. In contrast to recreational drugs, certain drugs are misused when used as performance enhancers. For example, students commonly misuse stimulant medications like amphet-amine (Adderall) in order to improve academic performance, or athletes may use this medication to improve athletic ability. (In addition to psycho-active drugs, which are the main focus of this text, performance-enhancing drugs such as anabolic-androgenic steroids, used by athletes to increase muscle mass and strength, are also considered drugs of abuse even though they are not used for psychoactive properties. Use of these steroids is considered unethical in professional sports, and they do carry side-effect risks.)

Another common term for a drug with the potential for abuse is "con-trolled substance." This is legal terminology for the substances that the government has designated to have abuse potential and that require con-trolled and monitored distribution in order to prevent this abuse. Con-trolled substances are divided into five drug schedules that categorize the drugs by their potential for dangerousness and addiction. These risks are weighed against their potential for therapeutic medical benefit. For exam-ple, Schedule I controlled substances are deemed to have no accepted medical use, and they are also deemed to have high potential for abuse. Schedule I drugs include cathinone, heroin, LSD, psilocybin, marijuana, and MDMA. According to federal law, none of these drugs can be pre-scribed legally. Schedule I drugs are some of the most likely to be sold as street drugs. (Of note, marijuana has become legal to purchase for medical or recreational use in several states, but federal law still prohibits its sale.) Schedule II drugs are also deemed to have high potential for abuse as well, but unlike Schedule I drugs, Schedule II drugs do have accepted medical use. Some examples of Schedule II drugs are amphet-amine drugs such as Adderall, methylphenidate (Ritalin), cocaine, fen-tanyl, oxycodone, and morphine. Drugs on schedules III-V are all deemed to have accepted medical use as well, and they are differentiated from one another in that the potential for abuse is said to decrease as one moves from Schedule II down to Schedule V. Prescribers can only prescribe drugs found on Schedules II–V, and each schedule requires different restrictions and standards for monitoring to ensure they are only prescribed for legitimate medical reasons. A drug's designated schedule is determined by recommendations from the DEA, which is part of the Department of Justice. The attorney general, who heads this department, has the final decision as to what drugs go on the list. Any controlled substance that is used illegally is called an "illicit" drug. This term includes completely illegal street drugs such as heroin or LSD, psychoactive prescription drugs used in an illegal manner not indicated by the prescriber, or even improperly used household substances such as inhalants. Another frequently seen term is "narcotics," which, despite its common usage, often has imprecise meanings. Currently, the DEA defines the word "narcotics" as synonymous with opioids. Historically, its precise legal and common definitions have varied. Commonly, it is used to mean any drug that is illegal, sold on the black market, and not used in medicine (essentially, any drug from Schedule I, including heroin, LSD, etc.).

The term "drug abuse" tends to connote that the activity is illegal. However, there are legal substances that are not generally considered "drugs" but nonetheless have high abuse potential. The two most common of such substances are alcohol and nicotine. For this reason, medical and mental health professionals do not currently have a diagnosis of drug abuse or drug addiction, but rather will diagnose a patient with having a substance use disorder and then note the specific substance. (For example, a patient might be given a diagnosis of opioid use disorder or alcohol use disorder.) In this way, the diagnosis avoids making a distinction between legal or illegal substance and between drug and nondrug substance. Instead, the focus is on the harmful use.

In the process of defining the terms above, an inescapable property of drug abuse itself becomes apparent. Drug abuse in the United States is situated on a fine line between two worlds: the medical world and the criminal world. Unlike illicit street drugs such as heroin, which is always illegal to possess, prescription drugs of abuse can be used either legally (medically) or illegally (recreationally). The health professions have one view of the nature of drug use, and the criminal justice system has a starkly different view. To a physician, a person who regularly uses heroin would be considered to have a disease or mental illness that ought to be treated, for example by referral to a methadone clinic. To a police officer, that same person would be considered a criminal because use and possession of heroin are illegal.

The key to understanding all of this is that psychoactive drugs in and of themselves are neither bad nor good, but rather it is the *context* of their use that makes the difference. When prescribed and used correctly, controlled substances can have great medical benefit. When used irresponsibly and inappropriately, these same controlled substances can be harmful. For example, if morphine pills are prescribed by a surgeon to be taken for a short time after an operation, this is considered legally and medically appropriate use. If the same morphine pills are handed out at a party for recreational use to people who are also drinking alcohol, the context has become dangerous, illegal, and nonmedical, and this would therefore constitute drug abuse. The importance of context in drug use is sometimes called "set and setting," referring to one's mindset and to the physical setting where the drug use takes place.

COMMONLY ABUSED PSYCHOACTIVE SUBSTANCES

In order to understand the scope of the problem with prescription drug abuse, it is useful to understand an overview of the broad scope of substance abuse in general, including legal and illegal psychoactive substances. Despite the sharp demarcation often made between prescription drugs and street drugs, the truth is that the chemical structures of many recreational drugs and many prescription drugs have similarities, and they often work by similar mechanisms and share similar effects. Some common recreational drugs of abuse are alcohol, marijuana, cocaine, heroin, MDMA (ecstasy), psilocybin (found in mushrooms), LSD, PCP, and methamphetamine. The three major classes of psychoactive prescription drugs of abuse are opioids, sedative-hypnotics (e.g., Xanax), and stimulants (e.g., Adderall).

As the similarities between certain prescription drugs and certain illicit drugs has become more appreciated by the general public, this has helped considerably to muddy the water for what constitutes socially and personally acceptable legal drug use versus stigmatized illegal drug use.

For example, on the prescription side of opioids, there are drugs such as OxyContin, Percocet, codeine, and fentanyl; and on the illegal drug side of opioids, the most commonly used drug is heroin. All opioids work by the same mechanism, and thus exhibit "cross-tolerability," so that withdrawal from one can be halted by use of another. The fact that heroin is essentially the same type of drug as the prescribed opioids has resulted in ever-increasing use of heroin by people who would never have considered using "drugs" in their life. Likewise, prescription stimulant drugs such as amphetamine (Adderall) and methylphenidate also have counterparts in the illegal world of stimulant street drugs, namely methamphetamine ("crystal meth"), MDMA (ecstasy), and cocaine in that they all have, at least in part, overlapping chemical properties, including the effect of acting as "uppers." Prescription sedative-hypnotics such as Xanax, Ativan, or Klonopin have effects on the body and chemical mechanisms that are most often compared with those of another nonprescription intoxicant: alcohol. This similarity is best illustrated in the case of alcohol withdrawal. For severe cases of alcoholism, a person develops physical dependence on alcohol such that they can experience tremors, nausea, vomiting, hallucinations, and more if they do not drink enough alcohol throughout the day. Alcohol withdrawal can even become deadly by resulting in seizures. To prevent a potentially deadly alcohol withdrawal, alcoholics must get "detoxed" in order to safely stop drinking. Alcohol detoxification usually involves administering sedative-hypnotics such as Ativan or Librium to patients in withdrawal to alleviate the withdrawal symptoms, since the chemical properties of those drugs are similar enough to alcohol. The Ativan or Librium is then slowly tapered off over several days while the body recovers from the physical dependence on alcohol. The illicit street drug PCP shares a similar chemical structure with the dissociative prescription drug ketamine. They are both members of a drug class called NMDA receptor antagonists. Ketamine is commonly used medically for anesthesia in emergency situations. It is also sometimes used by psychiatrists as an off-label treatment for refractory depression. Ketamine is sometimes illegally as a "club drug" for its dissociative properties.

Commonly used hallucinogens such as LSD and psilocybin have no currently approved medical uses, but renewed interest into possible medical uses of these substances has come about in recent years, and research into their benefit on mental health has been recently conducted. For example, a recent study by researchers at New York University and Johns Hopkins University investigated the effects of psilocybin on depression and anxiety in terminally ill cancer patients and found about 80% of psilocybin users in the study had clinically significant reductions in depression and anxiety lasting up to six months that allowed them to find a sense of peace in the face of their mortality.

Marijuana has seen significant drop in stigma in recent years as multiple states have legalized it for recreational use, and some states also allow it to be prescribed by doctors for medical use; for example, to treat chronic pain or to treat nausea associated with certain cancer treatments. The molecule cannabidiol was recently approved by the FDA to treat certain types of epilepsy.

MOTIVES FOR PRESCRIPTION DRUG ABUSE

The most common motives for initiating drug use are often different for prescription drug users versus street drug users. In general, some common motives people have for recreational drug abuse include obtaining a feeling of euphoria (a "high") and to dispel negative emotions. By contrast, among those who abuse prescription drugs, often the initial motive was not to get high but rather to treat the indicated medical or psychiatric symptom that prompted the prescription in the first place. For example, many people start using prescription opioids for legitimate pain relief, and only later after exposure to the drug does the motive for use switch to managing withdrawal symptoms, obtaining a feeling of euphoria, improving sleep, or dispelling negative emotions.

Given the sometimes similar effects between recreational and prescription drugs, and given that several Schedule I drugs—substances such as marijuana, psilocybin, and MDMA, which are legally deemed to have no acceptable medical application—are now seeing renewed interest by the medical and research communities as potential sources of new medications, it becomes clear that the worlds of prescription drugs and street drugs overlap more than one might expect. Part of this renewed interest in the research community stems from illicit use of these substances by various countercultural subgroups who have questioned the mainstream view that these substances have no therapeutic value. While there is not yet any scientific consensus on whether or not these substances truly do offer any net benefit that would outweigh the potential harms, the growing interest is illustrative of the idea that some users of street drugs may actually have been motivated to start using substances for the purpose of self-medicating conditions like physical pain, depression, and anxiety. The idea of self-medication is important in the study of substance abuse because some hypothesize that all addiction starts as a form of self-medication, but in the long run, the users find the strategy was maladaptive since they find themselves facing unintended consequences. For example, a person with anxiety and depression may start drinking alcohol as a way to take away the bad feelings for a while. However, if drinking alcohol becomes a person's main coping strategy to manage his or her emotions, this attempted self-medication quickly becomes an addiction. Another illustration of the way in which self-medication occurs is where some patients who become physically dependent on prescription opioids during the course of legitimate, appropriate pain treatment by their physicians can end up transitioning over to using street drugs such as heroin to maintain a physical dependency or to continue treating their pain. The problem with using street drugs for self-medicating is that they are not regulated by the FDA and have no guarantee of safety, quality, or purity. Drugs like heroin and cocaine are regularly cut with other powdery substances added in to dilute the drug, and sometimes these filler substances are harmful chemicals. Particularly with street heroin, the actual potency of the purchased drug can vary dramatically, because currently, heroin is often cut with a portion of fentanyl. Cutting heroin with fentanyl often results in bags of heroin that are much more potent than expected, since dealers rarely attempt to accurately convert the fentanyl dose to its equivalent heroin dose. Since fentanyl is up to 50 times more potent than heroin, the end result can be overdose death.

DISTRIBUTION PATTERNS OF PRESCRIPTION DRUGS OF ABUSE

By far, the most common way that prescription psychotherapeutics drugs are obtained and abused is through a bland, seemingly innocuous manner called diversion. in which prescription drugs are obtained from a friend or relative who has a legitimate prescription. For example, a college student with attention deficit hyperactivity disorder (ADHD) may give or sell some of her Adderall to her friends to use as a study aid or for the purposes of partying. Another example is a family member simply reaching into the medicine cabinet and taking an oxycodone tablet from another family member's bottle. Thus, as a result of diversion, 53.0% of misused prescription painkillers are obtained for free, given by a friend or relative. An additional 14.6% of prescription painkillers are also obtained via diversion from a friend or relative but by purchasing or stealing them instead of getting them for free.

Another way prescription drugs are obtained for abuse is simply through a prescription from a doctor. According to a 2014 survey by the Substance Abuse and Mental Health Services Administration (SAMHSA), 20.1% of painkillers used for nonmedical purposes were obtained from one doctor. Some patients obtain prescription drugs for nonmedical purposes by faking or exaggerating their pain symptoms in order to get pain medications they don't need. For example, a week's worth of prescription opioids may be prescribed to a patient for pain after a surgery. Then, at the follow-up visit with the surgeon, the patient may insist he is still in pain and needs more pain medications. In reality, the patient may or may not still be in pain, but the surgeon has no definitive way of knowing. Likewise, even if a patient does have legitimate pain, she could exaggerate the level of this pain, use some of her prescription for actual pain treatment, and then either divert extra pills she does not need or save them for later for recreational use. At encounters such as these, the doctor faces a dilemma: is the greater risk of harm to the patient to overprescribe the pain medications or to under-prescribe them? Instead of risking having a patient whose pain is untreated, the surgeon may instead prescribe another week's worth of pills. Since there is no truly objective way to know if a patient is in pain or not, there are often trends in how much doctors will prescribe opioids. In the 1990s, the popular mood among medical professionals was that doctors were too timid in prescribing opioids to patients with legitimate pain, and so prescriptions went up. In recent years, in light of increased prescription drug abuse, the new trend among doctors has been to prescribe less and less controlled substances. There are, however, also cases of dishonest medical professionals including doctors, nurses, and pharmacists as well who commit fraud. For example, a doctor may a write prescription for cash without a proper examination. A pharmacist may fill unfilled prescriptions a patient never picks up, charge the insurance company, and then sell the medication on the black market.

Another 2.6% of responders in the survey reported getting their pain medication from "more than one doctor." This represents an example of a phenomenon called doctor shopping in which patients may present to multiple doctors with the same complaint in order to get multiple prescriptions of the same medications. The extra prescriptions may be used for recreational purposes or be sold to street dealers for profit. Prevention of doctor shopping has improved over recent years with the introduction of statewide prescription monitoring databases available on the Internet, where the physician can check before writing a prescription and see if a patient has recently already been prescribed the medication by another doctor.

Unlike street drugs, most prescription drugs are not bought from a drug dealer. In fact, only 4.3% of prescription painkillers were obtained from a dealer or stranger. These dealers may obtain the prescription drugs in different ways. They may buy the medications from doctor shoppers. They may buy from patients who no longer use their prescriptions. For example, elderly people in retirement may sometimes supplement their incomes by selling their monthly bottle of prescription opioids or benzodiazepines. Dealers may also have a connection with a dishonest medical professional who can use his credentials to supply them with drugs, or they may sell drugs obtained by criminal methods, such as robbery of a pharmacy or of a vehicle transporting the prescription drugs.

When prescription drugs are bought off the street, it is not always known whether or not they are legitimate or fake. As mentioned previously, dealers sometimes sell counterfeit prescription pills that look like brand-name drugs such as Vicodin but in reality may contain illicit fentanyl or other substances.

TRANSITION FROM PRESCRIPTION USE TO STREET DRUG ABUSE

As has been shown in the above discussion, prescription drug abuse can occur when a legitimate prescription for a medical ailment transitions into an abuse of that same prescription drug. Likewise, given the often similar chemical structures, prescription drug abuse can then transition into abuse of street drugs.

Opioid drugs again give a good example for how prescription drug abuse can slide into abuse of street drugs. Opioid medications are among the most addictive substances that exist. The most commonly prescribed drug in the United States in 2016 was Vicodin, a combination pill that contains the opioid hydrocodone. Many stories exist of patients who break a bone or get surgery, develop excruciating pain, get prescribed a bottle of Vicodin or Percocet to treat the pain, and then inadvertently become hooked on opioids in the process. Suddenly, patients who had never abused drugs or alcohol before find themselves unable to stop taking the opioids. They may return to their doctor's office when the bottle runs out and insist the pain has not subsided and they require another month of medication. Then another month. And another month. Eventually, the doctor may decide the patient is exaggerating the pain and refuse to prescribe any more. However, by this time, the patient may be physically dependent on the drug, and may face withdrawal syndrome if the opioid is absent from their system for too long. Opioid withdrawal is very uncomfortable, causing patients to have several days of abdominal pain, nausea, vomiting, diarrhea, lacrimation (copious tears flowing from the eyes), tremors, anxiety, and agitation. Patients with chronic pain, such as nerve pain from a herniated lumbar disc, can also develop physical dependence on opioids by developing opioid-induced increased pain sensitivity, called hyperalgesia. As a result, their pain threshold decreases such that if they stop taking opioids, their baseline pain level from the herniated disc will actually be higher in the absence of opioids than if they had never taken the opioids in the first place. Many physicians by that point may become aware their patient has become addicted, and may continue to prescribe the opioids to help prevent the withdrawal and hyperalgesia. If the physician stops prescribing the opioids, the patient may then switch to another doctor in order to avoid the opioid withdrawal syndrome or hyperalgesia. If another doctor cannot be found to prescribe the medication, oftentimes the prescription medications can be purchased on the street from a drug dealer, sold in the same illegal way as marijuana or cocaine. Perhaps most surprisingly, it is not uncommon for patients who began taking opioid medications prescribed by their physician to eventually transition to one of the most stigmatized drugs in modern society: heroin. Often cheaper than its prescription opioid counterparts, heroin can sometimes provide a solution for a person addicted to prescription opioids who needs to maintain steady opioid supply. In this way, patients who would never have imagined taking heroin find themselves addicted. According to the CDC, about three out of four new heroin users report having abused prescription opioids prior to using heroin.

Mention of heroin often conjures familiar images of its use by stereotypical "junkies" in movies and on television: the yellowish-white powder is placed in a metal spoon with the handle curved underneath; a flame sparks from a cigarette lighter and heats the spoon from below; the powder melts and bubbles into an amber brown liquid; the brown liquid is drawn up through a needle into a syringe; a rubber tourniquet wraps around a user's arm just below the bicep; a vein pops up on the forearm; the needle is inserted into the vein; a red cloud of blood bursts into the surrounding amber sea as the syringe draws back; and a final push on the syringe pumps the mixture of blood and drug into the bloodstream, reaching the brain moments later; and the user slides down into a chair.

Typical heroin users are often depicted in the media as criminals and junkies who contribute nothing and spend their lives in and out of jail, committing crimes such as shoplifting or muggings to raise the money to get their next fix, with no other future in sight. Sadly, it is true that heroin use can cause a person's life to degenerate into such a downward spiral of crime and drug use. The end result of this downward spiral is often death by overdose. The body demands ever larger quantities of the drug to satiate its physical and psychological cravings, until one day the dose is too large and the user stops breathing. Given such frightening images of heroin abuse and the stereotypical and stigmatized addict who uses it, how it is that people end up transitioning to heroin from prescription opioids?

Many people who start taking prescription opioids for pain do not realize that these medications are in the same drug class as heroin. All drugs are essentially made of molecules, and what makes one drug different from the next is that each one is a unique molecular shape. Drugs are categorized into drug classes according to their function in the body and also based on their molecular structure, or shape. Much like OxyContin, morphine, codeine, and other commonly prescribed opioid drugs, heroin is a type of molecule called an "opioid" that has a very specific shape that allows it to interact with the body's brain and nervous system to produce effects such as pain relief and euphoria. Each different opioid medication consists of a different molecule with a unique shape. The fact that each opioid drug has its own unique shape allows it to interact with the body in its own unique way. Nevertheless, the molecular shapes of opioids and the effects of opioids are similar enough to each other that they comprise what is known as a family of drugs or a class of drugs. An analogy for this is how evolutionary biologists arrange animals into different classes. For example, birds or mammals are categorized as a "class" of animals, and within each class are multiple species that are distinct from each other but also have overall similar shapes and functions. For example, all birds have a similar shape, possessing such features as beaks, wings, and feathers, and yet the different species have slight differences that result in their interacting with the planet in different ways. Ducks have wings and can fly, but they also have webbed feet that allow them to spend much time swimming in lakes and ponds. The bald eagle also has wings to fly, but instead of webbed feet, it has strong eyesight and sharp talons, allowing it to perch on high trees, spot a distant fish, and swoop down to grab it. The different opioids are similar to each other in the same way. They all have a similar function biologically, but they are different in properties such as potency, rate of excretion from the body, level of euphoria, level of pain relief, and more. Once a person becomes addicted to prescription opioids and realizes heroin can be purchased with similar effect, the choice becomes much more palatable to them.

STIGMA AND THE PUBLIC PERCEPTION OF ADDICTION

Drug abuse and drug addiction are viewed with high levels of social stigma, meaning public perceptions of people with drug addictions are overwhelmingly negative. Stigma toward individuals with drug addiction indicates that they face great public mistrust, scorn, shame, prejudice, and discrimination.

To place the current levels of stigma against those with drug addiction into context, a comparison can be made to the stigma faced by those with mental illness in general. Historically, those suffering mental illnesses— such as depression, schizophrenia, post-traumatic stress disorder (PTSD), or bipolar disorder—have faced very high levels of stigma. In recent years, this stigma against mental illness in general has improved some-what. However, stigma against substance addiction remains very strong. For example, a 2014 survey at Johns Hopkins Bloomberg School of Public Health examined attitudes toward people with drug addiction. According to this survey, 90% of the respondents stated they would be unwilling to have a person with a drug addiction marry into their family, compared to 59% for a person with mental illness. Another 78% said they would be unwilling to have a person with a drug addiction work closely with them on a job. Nonetheless, despite the high rate of respondents who would not want a person with addiction in their family or at their job with them, 63% of respondents said discrimination against drug addiction is "not a serious problem." In terms of addiction treatment, 59% of respondents said it is ineffective, and 49% opposed increased government spending on drug addiction treatment.

Given the widespread stigma placed on drug abuse and addiction, it is difficult to understand the problem of prescription drug abuse without making a conscious effort to view addiction through a nonjudgmental framework. Remaining nonjudgmental is not always easy to do, and many readers will no doubt have personal stories or memories of family members or other figures in their lives who caused immense turmoil, dis-appointment, or even violence while under the influence of drug addiction or alcoholism. Drug use does not excuse crimes or poor behavior. At the same time, addiction is a true chronic disease in which actual changes occur in the brain, and therefore a purely moralistic view may not adequately address the problem.

It has been noted frequently that the stigma placed on addiction often contributes to difficulty in escaping it. If a person abuses and finds himself addicted, he will likely very much want to avoid the label of addict such as the heroin user described above. Once a person starts abusing drugs and become addicted, the desire to avoid the label of addict and the shame involved can actually work as an incentive to hide the addiction to maintain the image of a socially acceptable person. This denial and hiding of drug use can in turn negate the possibility of reaching out to friends and family for help or advice. In terms of prescription drug abuse, it may become easy for a person to hide her drug abuse behind the legal prescription, which appears to legitimize the addiction.

In order to help maintain a nonjudgmental framework when considering drug users, it is useful to recognize individuals' vastly different life experiences. For example, many people are surprised to discover that traumatic adverse childhood experiences (ACEs), which are essentially instances of childhood abuse, are shockingly more common than what is commonly believed. What is also clear from this study is that the rate of substance abuse later in life increases substantially with higher numbers of ACEs experienced in childhood. For example, according to the landmark Adverse Childhood Experiences (ACE) study published in 1997 by Felitti et al. in which nearly 10,000 adult medical patients were surveyed about adverse experiences in their childhoods, about 10% of people reported physical abuse as a child by an adult in the household who "often or very often hit you so hard that you had marks or were injured." Greater than one of every five people (22%) reported they had experienced childhood sexual abuse by an adult or person at least five years older. Specifically, 19.3% of respondents reported having their body touched or fondled in a sexual way during their childhood; 8.7% reported they were made to touch another person's body in a sexual way; 8.9% reported there was an attempt to have oral, anal, or vaginal intercourse with them during childhood; and 6.9% reported that an adult or person at least five years older actually had oral, anal, or vaginal intercourse with them. There were 25.6% of people reported living in a household with a person with substance abuse problems. There were 12.5% of patients whose mothers had been treated violently, and 3.4% of people had a household member go to jail. The study lists other types of ACEs as well. Patients who had at least one ACE were more likely to have had multiple ACEs, meaning multiple forms of abuse. Furthermore, the more ACEs a person had as a child, the more likely he or she was to have worse medical and mental health indicators and outcomes later in life. People with greater numbers of ACEs were more likely as adults to smoke cigarettes, have depression, have diabetes, and have heart attacks, and more. For the adult patients who had a history of zero ACEs, 1.2% had attempted suicide and 6.4% had used illicit drugs. For the adult patients who reported four or more ACEs during childhood (e.g., sexual abuse in addition to physical abuse and others), 18.3% had attempted suicide and 28.4% had used illicit drugs.

Clearly, from this study one can see that traumatic experiences increase one's likelihood of turning toward drugs of abuse, and this serves as an example of how maintaining a nonjudgmental frame of reference is useful in understanding drug abuse. The following quote by psychiatrist and trauma expert Dr. Bessel Van Der Kolk, MD, from his book *The Body Keeps the Score*, underscores the usefulness of the nonjudgmental frame toward substance abuse:

> We don't really want to know what soldiers go through in combat. We do not really want to know how many children are being molested and abused in our own society or how many couples—almost a third, as it turns out—engage in violence at some point during their relationship. We want to think of families as safe havens in a heartless world and of our own country as populated by enlightened, civilized people. We prefer to believe that cruelty occurs only in faraway places like Darfur or the Congo. It is hard enough for observers to bear witness to pain. Is it any wonder, then, that the traumatized individuals themselves cannot tolerate remembering it and that they often resort to using drugs, alcohol, or self-mutilation to block out their unbearable knowledge?

WHO ARE THE DRUG ABUSERS? DEMOGRAPHICS OF DRUG ABUSE IN THE UNITED STATES

To conclude the overview of prescription drug abuse presented in this chapter, it is necessary to have a broad snapshot of what sorts of people abuse drugs in the United States. Behind every statistic about drug overdose death, there is a real person who died and whose life had meaning. This person's death was not simply the death of a drug abuser, but rather the death of a daughter, a son, a brother, a sister, a best friend, a parent, or other connection. The following statistics demonstrate the ways drug abuse cuts across numerous demographic measures.

As might be deduced from the vast number of Americans who die from drug overdose each year, a vast number have used or abused drugs. In total, there were 323,148,000 people living in the United States in July 2016 according to the census website. Statistics about how many people abuse drugs—both illegal "street" drugs and psychoactive prescription drugs—have been compiled by SAMHSA. According to SAMHSA's report in 2016, about 130,628,000 of these people had used an illicit drug in their lifetime. This represents about 48.5% of the total population, which means that almost 1 out of every 2 people report to having used an illicit drug. Marijuana was by far the most used illegal drug, with 44% of people—nearly half the population—having tried it in their lifetimes. Nearly 1 in 10 people have used marijuana in the past month. Nearly 10% of people have tried LSD in their lifetimes. About 1 out of 50 people have tried heroin, about 1 in 20 people have tried methamphetamine ("crystal meth"), about 1 in 15 people have tried MDMA ("ecstasy" or "molly"), and about 1 in 7 people have tried cocaine. With 44% having tried marijuana, it is no wonder that several states have already passed laws to decriminalize it, whether by reducing penalties for possessing it to misdemeanor status, by allowing its use in a medically prescribed context, or by completely legalizing it for recreational use.

How frequently do people use illicit drugs? According to the same survey, 44,559,000 people aged 18 or older, or around 1 in 5 people, stated they had used illicit drugs during the past year, and 26,605,000 people from this age group, or around 1 in 10 people, had used illicit drugs in the past month. Around 1 in 14 people (7.1%) in this age group reported abusing prescription drugs during the past year, and about 1 in 40 people in this age group (2.4%), abused prescription drugs in the past month.

By Region

While 15% of people across the United States in 2016 said they used an illegal drug during the past year, there was notable regional variation in frequency of illegal drug use. The highest rate was in the Western region, with 19% of people having used an illicit drug in the past year. The lowest rate was in the South at 12.8%. The reasons for these variations are complex, but one of the biggest is that for the West Coast states, marijuana has become completely legal in Washington, Oregon, and California. Variations may also be cultural, with methamphetamine seen far less in the Northeast (0.1%) than in the South (0.2%) or west (0.5%).

By Ethnicity and Race

In terms of ethnic categories, Hispanic populations have a lower rate of lifetime usage, 37.3%, than non-Hispanic populations, 50.7%. (It should be noted here that "Hispanic" is not a racial category, but rather a distinct cultural marker showing a connection to numerous Spanish-speaking cultures. According to the U.S. Census, the term "Hispanic or Latino" refers to "a person of Cuban, Mexican, Puerto Rican, South or Central American, or other Spanish culture or origin regardless of race." Thus, a person who identifies as Hispanic may also identify as being from a certain race such as white, black, Asian, or Native American.)

Asians have the lowest lifetime rate of illicit drug use at 23.3%, followed by Native Hawaiians or other Pacific Islanders at 41.3%, blacks or African Americans at 46.0%, whites at 53.7%, two or more races at 57.7%, and American Indian or Alaska Natives at 58.7%.

By Urban versus Rural Setting

Rates of illicit drug use are similar in urban and rural settings. For example, 7.3% of people in large metropolitan areas reported misuse of prescription psychotherapeutics over the past month versus 5.2%.

By Education Level

Surprisingly, illicit drug use actually shows an overall increase among the more highly educated over the noneducated. For those aged 18 and older, the lowest rate of lifetime illicit drug use, 36.9%, occurred among those who had never graduated high school. The next lowest rate of lifetime illicit drug use, 47.9%, occurred among high school graduates. College graduates were the next highest at 53.3%, and the highest group were those with partial college completion or an associate's degree at 57.5%.

Not only do the rates of substance abuse differ according to educational level, but the types of drugs abused differ also. According to the National Institute of Drug Abuse, part of the National Institutes of Health (NIH), among college-age adults, defined as the age group of 19 to 22 years old, 7.8% used marijuana daily in 2016, compared to 4.0% in 1996. In all years, the prevalence was greater among those not in college than those in college. In 2016, of the non-college portion of this age group, 12.8% used marijuana daily, compared with 4.9% daily users in college. Alcohol use was higher in this age group in 2016 among those going to college, with 40.8% of college students having been drunk in the past month, compared with 30.4% of non-college students; and 9.9% of college students used Adderall in the past year compared with 6.2% of non-college students.

By Poverty Level

Increased poverty is associated with increased illicit drug use, but not as drastically as one might expect. Around 22.9% of the population below the poverty line reported illicit drug use in the past year, compared with 16.9% of the population with income twice that of the poverty line. This means about 1 in 4 people below the poverty line abuse illicit drugs in the past year, while about 1 in 6 people far above the poverty line abused illicit drugs in the past year.

By Gender

Males are more likely to abuse illicit drugs than females. About 55.1% of males greater than age 12 had used illicit drugs in their lifetime, compared to 45.8% of females greater than age 12.

By Employment Level

Those who are currently employed are less likely to have recently used illicit drugs than the currently unemployed. Illicit drug use over the past month included 9.4% of full-time workers, 10.2% of part-time workers, and 17.5% of the unemployed.

In Comparison to Alcohol Use

Patterns of alcohol consumption vary by age. For example, according to SAMHSA, in 2008, around 70% of Americans aged 21 have consumed alcohol within that past month. Among those in their thirties and forties, the average drops to around 60% who have consumed alcohol within the past month. This average drops again to around 40% for those 65 years old and above.

CHAPTER 2

The Science of Addiction and Drug Abuse

The push for increased opioid prescriptions starting in the 1990s resulted in more people than ever being exposed to addictive substances. These opioid medications were prescribed by physicians, and so they were not as likely to be viewed as being a moral failure (i.e., a deliberate choice to indulge in delinquent behavior). Suddenly, people who would otherwise never think of abusing a drug—even elderly people—found themselves addicted. Friends and family of these unexpected addicted people came to see that quitting an addictive substance is more than a matter of simply deciding to quit. As a result, a new wave of people began asking why is this happening, and what can we do about it? It has become clear that new and different solutions to the problems of drug abuse are needed, and therefore people are re-examining their understanding of the causes and nature of addiction.

Addiction and those who suffer from it have a long history of stigmatization. It is true that addiction and drug use are often associated with criminal behavior, violence, poor judgment, and recklessness. Most people throughout the world, no matter the context or culture, would like to see themselves and the ones they love live happy, healthy, and productive lives, according to whatever rules and norms the society enshrines. Therefore, they would understandably want to avoid the trouble that can follow people with addiction. Furthermore, in every civilization there is at some level the notion that people ought to master self-control in order to contribute best to the overall society. In the United States, for example, there is a tradition of "self-reliance" and "rugged individualism" in which everyone will live to their fullest potential and benefit the society most if they can rely on themselves. In religions such as Islam and Christianity, people are taught to varying degrees across different sects that intoxication is a sin because it clouds judgment and leads to further sins. Furthermore, on the strictly interpersonal, human level, it is painful to see loved ones ensnared in addiction (or mental illness in general). The idea of self-control is so central to the idea of personhood that it is almost like a death to see someone fall under the control of addictive substances. Much like an actual death, this sense of loss is often accompanied by a feeling of anger. At this point, many people ask, "why can't they just stop?"

When trying to account for the meaning of addiction, a common viewpoint is that addiction is a "moral failing," meaning that a conscious choice was made to give into temptation and to use the addictive substance. Another common viewpoint is that "addiction is a disease." Which viewpoint is correct? Truthfully, both are correct. Addiction clearly leads to moral failings (poor choices through poor judgment), and addiction is also clearly a disease. At their core, morals are simply rules a society has decided it will follow. These may be informal social norms, or they may be codified into law. Morals stem from historical sources such as religious and philosophical texts, and they stem from cultural and societal norms learned through social interactions with various people encountered throughout life. Without a doubt, intoxicants and addictive substances can alter cognition, meaning mental functions of the brain such as attention, decision making, planning, sensory perception, or calculation are altered. As a result of altered perception and cognition, these substances can alter people's judgment, meaning their conclusions about the world and decisions they take may be altered, which can lead to inappropriate behaviors. Furthermore, over time, addictive substances can lead to compulsion to use a drug, meaning a drive is developed in the brain to use the drug despite a conscious desire not to do so. As a result, these substances can play a role in people performing all levels of destructive and self-destructive acts including marital infidelity, poor job performance, killing oneself or someone else in a drunk-driving accident, stealing money to acquire more drugs, telling elaborate lies to hide one's addiction, and more. In this way, addiction causes people to fail to live up to even their own moral codes (which can be very distressing to them). And yet addiction is also clearly a disease in that addictive substances unquestionably cause structural changes to the brain and body that decrease self-control. These structural changes to the brain and body interact to keep people addicted, both by positive reinforcement (e.g., when opioid medication relieves pain and gives a sense of euphoria) and by negative reinforcement (e.g., when lack of opioid medication in a regular opioid user causes highly uncomfortable withdrawal symptoms).

Philosophically, confusion often arises in the debate about addiction due to what is known as a false binary. A false binary is a logical fallacy of "black-and-white thinking" in which a debate or concept is framed around two different positions that are falsely presented as though they are the "opposite." For example, cats and dogs are frequently discussed as being the opposite of each other, but strictly speaking, they are just two different species that have their own characteristics, and they are no more "opposite" each other than any other pair of species. Cats and dogs are not true opposites in the same way that north is the opposite of south or heads is the opposite of tails. In this way, the cultural debates about the nature of addiction present it as being either a) a controllable moral failing or b) an uncontrollable disease. However, there is no reason addiction has to be considered as strictly either one or the other. It can be both at the same time, or rather in the gray zone in between. Addiction causes people to lose control of themselves to varying degrees, as some people clearly have a more difficult time managing their addiction and staying in control than other people. This leads to a definition of addiction that is closer to its true nature: addiction is a disease of strong and habitual want that causes a person to have significantly less self-control and as a result leads to moral failings and harmful behaviors. The key notion is that control is less than normal but not completely absent. The fact that addiction is a disease does not mean that addicted people are not responsible for their actions. In fact, increasing self-control and relearning how to take responsibility for oneself are part of the treatment for addiction.

In order to better understand the struggles of people with addiction, it is useful to understand the psychological and physical (biochemical) changes that addictive substances cause, leading to psychological addiction and physical addiction.

PSYCHOLOGICAL ADDICTION AND CONDITIONING

A well-known effect of drugs of abuse is that they somehow cause a person to form a habit. What are habits, and where do they come from? Habits are patterns of behavior that are learned through repetition and that are often performed unconsciously. One of the most widely recognized habits is brushing teeth, which most people do ritualistically in the morning and evening without applying almost any conscious thought. Brushing one's teeth can occur in a state of being only partially awake, such as when one has just woken up in the morning or when one is about to fall asleep at night. Indeed, most people will be able to open the medicine cabinet or drawer, find their toothbrush, find the toothpaste, open the toothpaste, squeeze some on the toothbrush, brush their teeth on front and back, spit out the toothpaste, rinse, and put the toothbrush and toothpaste back in their places before they have even fully woken up in the morning! Clearly, habits are powerful phenomena in that we are not fully conscious of them but rather we simply perform them. In this way, they are somewhat like a behavioral program that our mind runs in response to certain stimuli. In terms of brushing our teeth, the stimulus or cue that our brain perceives is the very situation of waking up in the morning or also of going to sleep at night. When most people wake up or are about to go to sleep, the brain recognizes this scenario (e.g., by perceiving the amount of light outside, perceiving a person's level of sleepiness, perceiving what time it says on a clock) and it starts an automatic behavior to initiate the action of brushing teeth, largely encoded in the muscle memory.

At this point, many readers might rightfully ask, do habits really constitute an automatic behavior? The thought of people behaving in such a robotic, computer-like way can seem like an attack on the very ideas of personhood and free will. How automatic are habits, really? Does one not choose his or her own actions? It is clearly possible for a person to choose not to brush his or her teeth. However, again there is the risk of running into the logical fallacy of the false binary to assume the nature of behavior is an either/or choice between free will or automaticity. What has been shown is that *to a certain extent,* our actions and thoughts in response to stimuli are automatic. Another way to think of this is that the thoughts that arise in the conscious mind are not random, but they arise as a result of learned associations with thoughts currently in our minds or thoughts related to other objects we are currently sensing (seeing, hearing, etc.). For example, red traffic lights have become associated with the action of stopping a car, and so the thought comes automatically for most people to stop the car when a red traffic light is seen. Certainly someone could choose not to brush his teeth, but for most people, the idea that "perhaps I shall not brush my teeth this morning" never even enters their consciousness. Most people are used to brushing their teeth in the morning and associate the act of brushing teeth with the act of waking up so that they automatically do this. Furthermore, this person may also feel an internal urge to brush the teeth, since for many their mouth would feel unusual or dirty not to brush their teeth. Therefore, they are compelled by the urge to brush their teeth in addition to choosing to brush their teeth. It is also possible to imagine and "in-between state" in which someone "considers" not brushing their teeth, and may perform the habit more slowly, but ultimately follows the urge and completes the task. When we consider this example, perhaps then it is not such an unbelievable idea that at least some of our behavior is "automatic" in a certain way.

Addiction begins as a new habit, and habits are formed through a learning process called conditioning. This process was first demonstrated by Ivan Pavlov in the early 1900s in a famous experiment commonly known as Pavlov's Dogs. Pavlov was a Russian physician and scientist who investigated animal physiology to help better understand human physiology. He spent much time working with dogs and measuring their digestive fluids in order to understand how digestion occurs. He observed that the dogs began to salivate in the presence of food, which was not thought to be unusual. However, his greatest discovery was that over time, the dogs began to salivate not only at the sight of food, but eventually at the mere sight of the technician who brought them their food. He hypothesized that a learning had taken place and a new automatic behavior had been induced, causing "psychic salivation" in which the actual presence of food was not required for the dogs to mentally prepare for food. He then created an experiment where he was able to show it is possible to induce a behavior or mental state by the pairing of two stimuli, the unconditioned stimulus and the conditioned stimulus. The unconditioned stimulus in this case was the food, which was a natural and unlearned stimulus that caused the dog to salivate. For his conditioned stimulus, he chose a bell. He was able to create a behavior in the dogs by ringing the bell every time food was brought to the dogs. As a result, the dogs began to associate the bell with the food. After multiple feedings in the simultaneous presence of the bell ringing, the dogs began to respond to the ringing of the bell by salivating. This was therefore called a conditioned response. What had previously been a neutral stimulus, the ringing of the bell, was now a conditioned stimulus, because the dogs had gotten in the habit of hearing the bell when the food was coming. From this experiment, it becomes possible to hypothesize that certain "programmed" behaviors in humans might have similar origins. For example, a reasonable scenario to explain the origin of a person's habits such as teeth brushing might be that as a child, a conditioned response to brush the teeth was formed by the parent either offering reward for brushing teeth, such as praise, or offering punishment, such as scorn, for not brushing teeth. Likewise, most Americans who spent their childhoods in American public or private schools will be familiar with a form of Pavlovian conditioning very similar to the conditioning described above that was used in their own behavioral control: the school bell.

More modern experiments have been designed using conditioning to test the addictive potential of various drugs. For example, scientists sometimes use an experimental model called conditioned place preference. In this model, mice are placed in a closed environment (essentially a box) with multiple rooms for them to explore, and they are given a substance only in a certain place or room within this environment, and so the mouse learns to associate this particular place with the substance. If taking the substance was a rewarding experience in some way, the mouse will spend more time in the area where the substance was given.

Conditioning is the basis of a branch of psychology called behaviorism. A more specific name for the type of conditioning described above is classical conditioning. Other forms of conditioning exist as well, such as "operant conditioning." However, further in-depth explorations of operant conditioning, learning, and other behavioral concepts are beyond the scope of this book.

PHENOMENOLOGY OF ADDICTION

While it is correct that habits form a portion of the picture of how addiction functions, it is important to recognize that addictions are not merely habits. Habits are only one part of the full picture of addiction. The phenomenology of addiction—a description of addiction as it is experienced in the "first person"—is another helpful way to conceptualize the experience of addiction. For example, another way addictions cause people to change their behavior is through the formation of craving. Consider an even stronger urge than teeth brushing, a nearly irresistible urge that each person encounters on a daily basis: the urge to eat. Whereas brushing your teeth can be performed almost absentmindedly, without giving it much thought or noticing it much, people are compelled to eat primarily by a feeling they have, the feeling of hunger. When most people skip a meal, or especially if they skip two or more, the craving to eat takes over an ever-greater portion of their consciousness. Their attention and consciousness become ever more focused on the acquisition of food. Their mood becomes irritable. The content of their thoughts becomes increasingly filled with images of food and plans to acquire food. Indeed, one can begin to remember the taste of food so well as to "almost taste it." In response to this mental state, habits are activated, and a person's actions will become more geared toward finding food. For any reader who does not believe this, attempt not eating for an entire day except water and see how much your thoughts turn to food and see how much mental effort it will take not to eat anything. (Of course, this challenge excludes those who would not, for medical reasons, safely skip a meal.) For those who attempt this, or for those who can remember a similar instance in their lives, it will have become apparent that willpower (the mental capacity to resist urges) only lasts so long in the quest to not eat food.

So what is "hunger" and how is it able to control the thoughts? Hunger can be thought of as a "mental state" or "state of consciousness." Other common states of consciousness that people experience on a regular basis include sleepiness, thirst, fear, and others. All of the molecular mechanisms of hunger are not known, but what can be shown is the existence of certain hormones such as ghrelin and other molecules that are released in the bloodstream when the gastrointestinal tract in empty and the body needs more nutrients. These hormones act on the brain to alter the motivation of the person to seek food.

Thus far, several examples have been presented of common automatic behavior in humans. The first major type was the common habits people perform such as brushing one's teeth in the morning and at nighttime. The second major type of automatic behavior involved having one's mental faculties become increasingly focused on the obtainment of food in relation to increasing hunger. Understanding these two familiar automatic behaviors and acknowledging the existence of such behaviors in all people, including the reader, is the first stepping-stone toward empathy for and understanding of the plight of the addicted individual. Addictive substances are addictive because they involve the formation of habits and cravings that cause the addicted individual to behave in ways they cannot always control. In fact, addiction has much in common with any rewarding behavior. The reason that addiction is separate and more problematic than the automatic behaviors described above is that addictive substances chemically and anatomically alter the reward mechanism circuitry in the brain, which can lead to self-destructive changes in behavior.

Understanding the brain's reward system is crucial to understanding the development of craving in addiction. Addictive substances all have one trait in common, and that is they produce a feeling called euphoria. In normal life, when we have a good experience, our brains reward us with dopamine, and we "feel good." Euphoria is that same feeling, mediated by the same dopamine release, and extends it out through time. Addictive substances all make the person feel good and indeed, genuinely happy when he or she first takes them. (Much in the same way children feel good when getting praise from their mothers.) The problem with addictive substances is that the "good feeling," or euphoria, is not elicited from a natural stimulus or interaction with the world, but rather by a chemical reacting in the brain. People want to feel good, especially people who have had difficult lives, and so they seek more of this feeling. The drug has become what the mother's praise was, a release of dopamine into the reward circuitry. However, the mother's praise was given for self-beneficial behavior, clean teeth, and the hunger pangs led to the acquisition of nourishment. Addictive substances chemically stimulate the reward center, and so the brain learns to seek out more of the substance. Thus, not only does a habit form, but also the urge and craving for the substance form.

It is now clear how the behaviors of people suffering from addiction relate to behaviors every person experiences in their own lives every day. The question arises: So what? If a person becomes addicted, forms a habit of using the substance in certain scenarios (e.g., at a party), and the person develops urges and cravings for the substance, then what is the problem? If they can just take more of the drug to satisfy the craving, why does it matter if someone becomes addicted to a drug? Given that euphoria is by definition a good feeling, and particularly given that many people have led difficult lives and haven't experienced much good feeling before or felt much love, what is wrong with letting them take drugs that make them feel good? Some of the reasons include a) drugs can have deleterious side effects such as overdoses; b) the use of drugs and the time and money spent in their attainment often come at the expense of time better spent maintaining one's social interactions, jobs, and financial security; c) transmission of infectious diseases among users of shared needles; and d) harm to physical health caused by impurities in many street drugs.

How is it that addictive substances make the transition from one-time rewarding event to a recurring habit and then up to full-blown cravings and urges? The answer has to do with the chemical properties of the drugs and their effects on the brain.

BIOCHEMICAL CAUSES OF ADDICTION

To understand exactly how addiction affects the brain chemically, it is useful to have a broad understanding of how the brain is organized and to understand the structure and function of certain parts of the brain that are particularly important in understanding addiction. In order to discuss the brain structure, it is useful to have a basic understanding of the levels of organization of the physical structure of the human body, from the macroscopic level of the whole organism all the way down to the microscopic level of cells and molecules. It is well known that all matter is composed of atoms, and thus the human body is composed of atoms. Atoms combine to form collections of atoms called molecules. Under certain conditions (such as the environmental conditions here on earth), molecules can combine and arrange themselves in ways so as to form cells, which are the basic unit of life. A well-known molecule found in cells is DNA, which contains the genetic code. The human body is composed of trillions of cells. These cells of the human body are differentiated into multiple different types, such as fat cells or red blood cells. Groupings of different cell types are arranged into four types of tissues. These tissue types are muscle, epithelial (works as a lining, for example, the outer layer of skin), connective tissue (such as in bones or cartilage), and nervous tissue (such as in the brain or spinal cord). Different tissue types combine to form organs, such as the brain, the heart, the liver, the kidney, etc. Different organs are arranged to form different organ systems. For example, the digestive system is composed of the mouth, the esophagus, the stomach, the small intestine, the liver, the pancreas, the gallbladder, and the large intestine, all of which work together to digest food. All the organ systems combine to make the organism, which is the individual human. Thus, the body of each person is like a vast, complex ecosystem of different structures all working together across different orders of magnitude to form an integrated whole, with atoms forming molecules, molecules forming cells, cells forming tissues, tissues forming organs, organs forming organ systems, and organ systems forming the whole organism. Small changes at the atomic or molecular level can and often do cause whole organism changes. For example, at the atomic level, the amount of sodium in the blood drastically alters the distribution of water in the body, such that if there is a drop in the blood sodium level, water will leak from the blood vessels into the surrounding tissues, causing the face, arms, legs, and indeed the whole body to swell up. This type of swelling can sometimes be seen in athletes after vigorous exercise when they sweat out too much sodium in the form of salt. Another example from the microscopic world that results in vast changes in the organism is a process called *molecular signaling*. The occurrence of molecular signaling is the basis of most medications as well as street drugs. Molecular signaling occurs when a molecule travels though the body, such as through the blood, then encounters a cell, and then causes a change in the cell. A molecule such as the drug pseudoephedrine (Sudafed) can travel to cells in the nose and tell these cells to stop having an allergic reaction to pollen. Soon, that person's sneezing and runny nose will cease. How can a molecule cause sneezing and runny noses to go away? One feature of all cells is that they contain receptors. Receptors are like keyholes in the structure of a cell, often made of proteins. When a molecule with the correct shape encounters a receptor, it can "unlock" a function of a cell, much like a car key with the correct shape can cause a car's motor to turn on. An example of how this works is how the drug pseudoephedrine, which is essentially just a molecule that has a very specific shape, can decrease nasal congestion. When pseudoephedrine molecules reach the tiny blood vessels that around the nasal passages, these molecules encounter receptors—"keyholes"—on the cells that comprise these blood vessels. These receptors fit the specific "key" shape of the pseudoephedrine molecules. Changes at the receptors result in further changes inside the cell, and in this case, the cell stops producing mucus. This process of molecular signaling—with molecules interacting with receptors to cause changes in the cell function—is the same process by which most drugs work in the body, whether prescription drugs or street drugs. Different drugs work in this or that part of the body because different cell types contain different receptors. The cells in the heart have different receptors than cells in the brain, and this is why some medications work for heart problems and other medications work for the brain.

Broadly, the brain is composed of cells called neurons surrounded by supportive cells called "glial cells." The neurons are the "stuff" of the brain, and the existence of neurons differentiates nerve tissue from other types of tissues. Neurons are a special type of cells that can send messages to each other and different parts of the body through electric conductance. The nervous tissue is arranged to form organs of the nervous system. The nervous system is composed of a central nervous system, which consists of the brain and the spinal cord, and a peripheral nervous system, composed of peripheral nerves. Peripheral nerves extend from the spinal cord to the rest of the body and are about the size of an electrical cord at the point where they leave the spinal cord. These nerves split and branch like tree branches as they leave the spinal cord and reach their destination at various points in the body, extending out like thin wires connecting the brain to various muscles, areas of skin, and more. The function of the central nervous system is to process or interpret sensory information that comes from the peripheral nervous system, and then based on that information, initiate an action that is carried out by the peripheral nervous system. For example, peripheral nerves that innervate the skin are able to sense temperature, pain, texture of surfaces, etc., and so if someone is outside and the temperature is very hot from being in the sun, the peripheral nervous system senses this hot temperature, relays this information to the brain at the sensory cortex, and a decision is made to move to the shade; and thanks to visual information at the occipital cortex, the brain can initiate action to move toward the shade, an electrical signal is sent from the motor cortex of the brain to the leg and arm muscles, and the person walks to the shade.

Of note from this example, it is already clear that the brain itself is organized into different functions that are often located at different physical locations on the brain. The largest part of the brain is called the cerebrum, which is responsible for generally higher functioning and higher complexity tasks such as planning, imagining, language, logic, and more. The motor cortex, responsible for motor function such as running or lifting, is located on the left side of the cerebrum just behind the midline. Below the cerebrum is the midbrain, which contains structures such as the hypothalamus (controls multiple hormones), the thalamus (relays sensory information from the peripheral nervous system to the central nervous system), the amygdala (plays a role in fear), and the hippocampus (plays a role in memory formation). These structures are somewhat more primitive and are associated with such phenomena as emotion, stress, and memory. Below the midbrain is the brainstem, which contains even more primitive (yet extremely crucial) functions such as control of breathing. Finally, attached to the brainstem is the cerebellum, a "fine tuning" portion of the brain that coordinates the movements of several muscles to produce smooth movement.

At the anatomical and molecular level, the brain processes rewards in a structure called the "mesolimbic dopamine circuit." Any type of reward, whether intellectual accomplishment, enjoying a football game, or eating a delicious snack, is accompanied by a release of dopamine in this neural circuit. For this reason, the mesolimbic dopamine circuit is often called "the final common pathway of reward."

Now that a basic understanding of all the relevant structures of the brain has been covered, it is possible to understand ways in which addiction affects the brain down to the structural and molecular level. Again, this is so important because drugs are essentially different types of molecules, and our main interest is how do these molecules affect the whole organism in such a way as to cause addiction. The common factor that all forms of addictive drugs share is that they directly act upon the brain's reward pathway, the mesolimbic dopamine circuit, to cause the brain cells to release a larger-than-natural burst of dopamine. Thus, the brain interprets the presence of these drugs as a source of good things. The more reward that is derived from behaviors, the more the brain will seek to perform those behaviors. Thus, the brain learns that drugs are the ultimate source of reward and good feeling, and therefore more time and effort need be spent to acquire this drug.

What is special about addictive drugs that they have this ability to trigger this burst of dopamine? What is it about addictive drugs that the mesolimbic dopamine circuit loves so much that it wants to reward someone for using the drugs? The answer is that the molecules found in drugs of abuse have structures that are similar to molecules our own bodies produce. One way to think about this is that the human body produces "its own drugs." The effect-producing molecules found in opioids, alcohols, cannabis, benzodiazepines, and other drugs mimic molecules that are produced by our own bodies. For example, in the same way that the cells in the seeds of a poppy plant produce small amounts of the opioids morphine and codeine for their own molecular signaling, our brains produce their own opioids called endorphins. Endorphins have similar structures to morphine, heroin, and other opioids. The name endorphin was even created by combining the words "endogenous" and "morphine," hence meaning something like "morphine originating from within the organism." Endorphins are excreted by the body to help decrease pain and can also produce euphoria. A common example of both functions of endorphins is their release during aerobic exercise such as running. During exercise, endorphins are released, which helps decrease the pain involved with running so that the person can run longer. Likewise, the person is rewarded for running and can gain a "runner's high" by direct activation of the mesolimbic reward system by the endorphins. Therefore, due to the existence of these self-made opioids, cells in our brain's reward pathway and other parts of our nervous system directly contain opioid receptors. Thus, when opioids originating from outside the body are introduced into the body at amounts higher than what the brain would naturally receive, the brain views this as an incredibly positive development. The entire episode becomes vividly remembered by the brain as an important event, and thus memory of taking the drug is strongly encoded in the brain, the environment where the drug was taken is encoded along with the memory of the drug, and multiple other aspects of the scenario in which the drug was taken are strongly encoded into memory. In this way, addictions change the structure of the brain in terms of how neurons connect to each other, because a learning takes place. This is not so different from any type of learned behavior, which always is accompanied by strengthening or weakening of neural connections in response to positive or negative associations.

PHYSICAL ADDICTION AND DEPENDENCE

Addiction involves both drug abuse and drug dependence. Drug abuse is using a drug in a way that's risky, irresponsible, and potentially dangerous. Drug dependence implies a physical dependence on the drug that causes a person to continue taking it in order to avoid withdrawal. Abuse can be thought of as the pleasure-seeking aspect of the addiction. People use drugs despite the risk because they gain a reward feeling for doing so, and in this way the drugs offer a positive reinforcement, aka the "carrot." Dependence can be thought of as the negative reinforcement, aka the "stick," in that it causes people to take the drug not because the drug gives them euphoria, but because they will suffer a withdrawal if they do not take the drug.

Drug abuse can include a one-time instance of risky use drug. In the context of prescription drugs, drug abuse includes using the drug in a manner outside of what the doctor prescribed. Binge drinking is a common example of alcohol abuse. If a group of students who go to a party once every week or two and "drink to get drunk," they are usually engaged in binge drinking. People often binge drink in order to feel the euphoric effects of alcohol and to reduce social inhibition. However, the behavior is risky. Binge drinking causes the blood alcohol level to rise to a level so high that cognition becomes severely impaired. Subsequently, the drinker can be said to have lost control of their behavior because their behavior becomes increasingly contradictory with decisions they would make if their judgment wasn't impaired. Risks involved with binge drinking include injury from falls, motor vehicle accidents from drunk driving, contracting sexually transmitted diseases, increased risk of suicide, unintended pregnancy, violence toward others, and interpersonal problems between friends and families over things said while intoxicated.

Drug dependence involves changes to the brain and nervous system that will cause the dependent person to have physical withdrawal symptoms if the body is deprived of the drug. Alcohol dependence is the most dangerous type of drug dependence because if an alcohol-dependent person suddenly stops drinking alcohol, he or she will experience alcohol withdrawal, which can result in death. When someone becomes addicted to alcohol to the point where they start drinking it every day in increasing quantities, they start to build drug tolerance. Dependence always occurs in the context of increased tolerance of a drug. Simply put, tolerance is when the body requires ever-increasing amounts of a drug in order to achieve the same effect. Someone who takes heroin for the first time will need less of the drug to get high than someone who has been taking heroin daily for many years. What occurs is that the user requires more and more of the drug to obtain the same high as they felt the first time they took it. After the body and brain are bombarded by the heroin on a regular basis, the body seeks to reestablish its natural resting equilibrium, and so the brain and nervous system become desensitized to a certain extent. Cells can respond to this constant bombardment by having the opioid receptors become less sensitive to the presence of heroin. In some cases, cells may also decrease the number of receptors available. The mesolimbic dopamine circuit, the reward system of the brain, begins to view the presence of the drug as normal and no longer responds by secreting the dopamine that gives the reward feeling of euphoria. This is somewhat analogous to what it's like to jump into a cold swimming pool on a hot day. At first, the swimmer might feel the water is extremely cold, possibly even shivering. "Cold" is a sensation detected by the nervous system via temperature-sensing nerve endings located at the skin. After several minutes, the swimmer's body often adjusts and he or she gets used to the temperature, no longer feeling as cold. As long as the water is not extremely cold to the point where it could cause bodily damage, the nervous system will recognize that continued awareness of the cold is not useful and will decrease the transmission of the signal for "cold" to the brain. Another example of tolerance occurring in the nervous system is the way it filters out background noise. Imagine sitting in the kitchen and reading a book. All of a sudden, the refrigerator stops humming. Prior to the stopping of the humming fridge, most people would not have even noticed that the sound of the refrigerator running was even there. The brain filters out that sound because it is sensed to be merely background noise. Even though the sound signal is constantly present and being sensed by the ears, it does not enter into conscious awareness because it does not change and is not useful to be aware of. No attention is given to it. Similar to this, when the mesolimbic dopamine circuit is bathed in heroin for a long time, it becomes habituated to the drug's presence and no longer finds it useful to transmit the signal of reward to the rest of the brain.

When the presence of heroin becomes as unremarkable to the brain as does the hum of a refrigerator, this is clearly a problem. If the body thinks that the new normal state of affairs is having a steady stream of heroin filling its opioid receptors, what happens when the stream of heroin suddenly stops flowing? The answer is a state of highly unpleasant affairs called withdrawal.

In order to understand withdrawal, it is imperative to first discuss a little more about the overall effects of drugs on the body. So far, we have only discussed how substances of abuse affect the mesolimbic dopamine circuit—the brain's reward circuit—as this circuit is crucial to understand as the basis for how addiction and abuse begin. However, in addition to the brain's reward circuit, neurons extend through the body, and so opioid receptors also exist throughout the body and cause a multitude of effects. As a result, receptors across the whole body, not just in the brain, gain tolerance at the same time. Heroin and other opioids have effects in the body beyond just euphoria. Opioids cause the pupils to constrict. Opioid receptors in the gastrointestinal tract cause it to slow down (thus, constipation is a side effect of opioids). They play a role in transmitting the feeling of pain to the brain. They slow the movement of muscles and cause deep relaxation. They cause the rate of breathing to go down. They cause dry mouth and cause the tear ducts to release less tears. Through increased use, the body eventually gains tolerance against these side effects in the same way that the brain did, through desensitizing receptors and decreasing the overall amount of receptors.

Withdrawal—caused by removing the steady stream of drug from a person's body—would be bad enough if it only involved the brain, but the full body involvement makes it truly terrible. Withdrawal from a substance can be conceptualized as a change in the physiologic state of the body that is similar to the opposite effect of whatever the substance had done to the body originally. Withdrawal from each drug is different depending on how the drug affects the body, and so each has a characteristic withdrawal syndrome. So what does opioid withdrawal look like? Essentially like the opposite of the effects discussed above. Instead of a feeling of euphoria, a person in withdrawal will have a feeling of dysphoria (negative mood state), anxiety, and/or irritability accompanied by intense cravings. These cravings are analogous to the cravings one would experience for food or water in a state of deprivation of either. The consciousness becomes consumed with thoughts of obtaining more of the drug to satiate the reward center. The person in withdrawal from opioids is much like an airplane pilot who crashed in the desert, with sun blazing in the sky, and crawls dehydrated across the dunes, pleading, "Water! Water!" Compounding the mental anguish of this withdrawal is the intense bodily discomfort. The pupils dilate and lights become painfully bright. The gastrointestinal tract becomes overactive, resulting in diarrhea, abdominal cramps, nausea, and vomiting. Tears stream from the eyes, and mucus runs from the nose. The bodily relaxation disappears and is replaced by restlessness and tense muscles. The tiny hairs across one's body stand up straight, resulting in prominent "goosebumps." (Goosebumps are caused by microscopic muscles in the skin called piloerectors that make the hairs stand up.) A feeling of discomfort and restlessness spreads throughout the arms and legs, an almost electrical feeling, and this causes a person to constantly get up from their seat and pace around in an attempt to evade the bodily discomfort that permeates everywhere no matter how they position themselves. (Discomfort and comfort are feelings. Feelings are a product of the nervous system. Therefore, if opioids acting on the nervous system can produce a feeling of comfort, it is also plausible that in withdrawal, a person would feel this sort of uncomfortable, electrical feeling throughout.) These symptoms do not go away quickly. Symptoms are the worst during the first week but typically last about a month. Some symptoms last longer than a month. This whole period of withdrawal in which the drug is allowed to completely exit the system is also called detoxification, or "detox" for short, as the process of withdrawal also denotes the process of removing the drugs (which have toxic effects) from the body. The process of withdrawal from opioids is miserable. It is so miserable that longtime users often remain on opioids more to avoid withdrawal than because they are actually deriving any pleasure from taking the drugs. Other substances can have even worse withdrawal symptoms, and alcohol withdrawal is actually life-threatening due to the occurrence of a state called delirium tremens as well as the risk of alcohol-withdrawal seizures. To help those with physical substance dependence to make withdrawal symptoms more tolerable and to help avoid any life-threatening risks, patients can go to "detox centers" and be given medications to help taper off their substances of abuse. Typically, these centers offer several days to a week of methadone for opioid withdrawal or several days to a week of benzodiazepines for either alcohol or benzo withdrawal.

PSYCHOLOGICAL DEPENDENCE

Sadly, even after the acute detoxification period is over, for most people who have become addicted, they will never be able to return to a completely normal state of affairs like before they had started the substance of abuse. Changes in the brain have already occurred, and so though a person may no longer be physically dependent on the drug, he or she will usually forever to a certain degree be psychologically dependent on it.

What does it mean to be psychologically dependent on a substance versus physically dependent? Physical dependence is the scenario described above in which physiologic changes to the body occur so that the person will be physically ill (and in the case of alcohol, will possibly die) without the presence of the addictive substance. Psychological dependence involves the presence of 1) learned behaviors that can be set off by numerous environmental triggers in a person's life and environment that will cause them to want to take a drug, and 2) an altered baseline mood and sense of well-being.

Environmental triggers are individual to each person and are essentially various instances of conditioning that will cause a person to desire to take a drug. Much like the children at school who have been conditioned to pack up their books and move on to the next class at the sound of the bell, or like the how the "ping" sound on a cell phone of a text message arriving causes most people to have an irresistible urge to check their phone, individuals who have become addicted to drugs will also have become conditioned to respond to other neutral stimuli that were present at the time of the drug use. Psychological dependence is much like what occurred with Pavlov's dogs when they were conditioned to associate the ring of the bell with the arrival of food. The bell became a trigger that cause the dog to salivate and become very hungry. When the addicting chemical effects of drugs were described earlier, the discussion mostly involved the chemical effect of the drugs binding to receptors on the brain's reward systems, that is, the mesolimbic dopamine circuit. However, clearly a person is more than just the effects of his or her mesolimbic dopamine circuit. When a person takes an addictive drug, this drug is taken by an actual individual person in an actual individual place. Any person, place, or thing that is regularly part of the environment where the addictive drug is taken can serve as a trigger for the drug use. The result of an environmental trigger can depend on the individual person's inclination level of addiction and also the length of time a person has been away from the addictive substance. The trigger can encourage the drug use both by the initiation of a habit and also by the initiation of intense cravings that fill the mind and cause it to minimize other goals. For example, imagine a former alcoholic (arbitrarily male in this example) who drives by a former bar he used to frequent. Even if a long time has passed since he has gone to this bar, the mere sight of it can trigger a desire to drink. Depending on the person, his level of addiction, and his level of impulse control, he may or may not be able to overcome the urge to go have a drink.

What is the nature of this psychological dependence in terms of brain function? How do habits form in the brain, and what makes them so difficult to ignore for some people? In addition to the physiologic changes in receptor concentrations caused by addictive substances that trigger the reward system in the mesolimbic dopamine circuit, the habits formed by addictions can be conceptualized multiple different ways. In one way, we can describe these bad habits as maladaptive coping strategies. This involves a person learning an ultimately detrimental strategy for dealing with stressors. For example, a person might learn that when she is feeling stressed, she ought to reach for a drink, as this will surely decrease her anxiety level. However, this is ultimately a poor strategy in the long run because it merely blunts the anxious feeling instead of addressing the cause of the stress. Maladaptive coping strategies can be altered theoretically through therapy in which a person incrementally learns more mature and healthy coping strategies that afford more self-control.

IMPULSIVITY-COMPULSIVITY

Another, more difficult to treat, form of psychological dependence that can form in addiction is when it progresses to one of many types of impulsive-compulsive disorders. The concepts of impulsivity and compulsivity are crucial to understand to get at the nature of psychological addiction as they both represent ways in which the conscious mind loses control. In fact, understanding impulsivity and compulsivity can help in understanding multiple different mental illnesses that are all linked to issues of difficulty controlling habits. Examples of common impulsive-compulsive behaviors are attention-deficit hyperactivity disorder (ADHD), compulsive Internet use, compulsive shopping, hypochondriasis, obsessive-compulsive disorder (OCD), and trichotillomania (a disorder in which people cannot stop pulling their hair out). Impulsivity involves the brain having difficulty saying no to the initiation of an action. Therefore, impulsive people act before they think in order to satisfy an urge to gain an immediate positive reward feeling. This is often noted, for example, in children with ADHD. Compulsivity involves the brain performing a behavior having difficulty saying no to the continuation of an action. Thus, compulsive actions are performed because they are an urge to relieve a negative feeling, and thus people cannot stop once they have started. Both impulsivity and compulsivity result in a person having a decreased self-control.

A common nonaddiction example of impulsivity and the brain having difficulty saying no to an action is seen in children with ADHD. These children are noted to have difficulty staying focused on one task and will impulsively leap from one activity to the next, whichever appears to offer the greatest immediate gratification (which correlates with greatest release of dopamine from the mesolimbic dopamine circuit). Thus, they have difficulty focusing on one task and delaying gratification. Gambling addiction is another example of poor impulse control. Gambling can involve winning a relatively large amount of money at one time. When money is won in this quick way, it can cause a quick burst of dopamine release in the reward circuitry. Indeed, impulsivity often involves participation in risky behavior since the immediate reward is often high. Because the impulsive brain acts in a way to seek quick rewards, it has trouble avoiding the initiation of this behavior once it is triggered environmentally. Impulsivity is subject to positive reinforcement, in that the more times a person is exposed to a rewarding stimulus, such as the presence of an addictive drug, the less inhibited a person becomes toward that stimulus and the more impulsively she or he will indulge in that stimulus. As might be expected, risk of addiction is higher in people who have natural, preexisting conditions of decreased impulse control, such as with ADHD, mania in bipolar disorder, or borderline personality disorder.

A common non-addiction example of compulsivity is seen in obsessive-compulsive disorder. The most well-known example of compulsive behavior in OCD is a person who cannot stop repetitively washing his or her hands. This compulsive handwashing is the result of an irresistible urge, an uncomfortable, negative, anxious feeling of being dirty that will not go away unless the person performs the compulsive behavioral "program" of handwashing. Thus, compulsion differs from impulsive behavior, which seeks to obtain feelings of mental reward, while compulsive behavior seeks to escape feelings of mental punishment. Once the program has been started, both the impulsive and the compulsive person may have awareness that the behavior is ultimately detrimental, and yet due to brain circuitry, they are unable to modify their behavior to a great extent. Compulsivity is subject to negative reinforcement in that the more often a behavior is performed that relieves a negative state (such as a hunger, a craving, or a withdrawal state), the more easily and automatically the behavior will be initiated.

In summary, impulsivity and compulsivity are both types of urges that compel a person to perform an action, the difference being that impulsivity involves an urge to obtain a reward feeling and compulsivity involves an urge to relieve a negative feeling. Of note, all habits, including ones as mundane as brushing one's teeth, are in effect mild compulsions, though the urge to perform average habits is not as difficult to stop as the urge to perform a compulsion as seen in OCD.

Given that most people are not completely impulsive or compulsive all of the time, what keeps a person able to avoid acting out these urges? Again, science can offer a model for understanding. Though the following is a very simplified presentation of what occurs in the brain, it allows for an adequate initial understanding of problems addicts face at the level of the brain. Essentially, in all impulsive-compulsive disorders, including drug addiction, an imbalance occurs between the parts of the brain that inhibit undesirable behaviors and the parts of the brain that urge undesirable behaviors. Everyone faces multiple urges at all times, such as urges to eat, urges to urinate, urges to scratch an itch, urges to check e-mail or text messages, and so on. However, different people have different abilities to inhibit these urges and not act on them. Various urges constantly spring forth in a person's consciousness, and these urges are related to the stimuli around a person. From these urges, a person then selects the urge she or he wishes to act upon and inhibits the others. Therefore, action-outcome of thought is selected as intersection between the inhibitory functions of the brain and the urge functions. The area of the brain mostly involved with the reward-seeking, positive-reinforcement urges of impulsivity is called the ventral striatum, and it may come as no surprise that the ventral striatum actually contains the mesolimbic dopamine circuit and mediates its interaction with the rest of the brain. The area of the brain mostly involved with the punishment-avoiding, negative-reinforcement urges of compulsivity is called the dorsal striatum. The area of the brain most involved with inhibition of these urges is called the prefrontal cortex. In this way, the action-outcome of thought is essentially the intersection of the inhibitory function of the prefrontal cortex and the motivational urges of the ventral striatum and the dorsal striatum.

TREATMENT OF ADDICTION

Given the multiple ways that addictive substances alter the brain through intertwined chemical, anatomical, and psychological mechanisms, it is not surprising that treatment for addiction is quite difficult.

Addiction is best thought of as a chronic disease, in that it is generally never completely cured, but rather it is managed over the lifetime. For example, another common chronic disease is type 1 diabetes, which involves high levels of sugar in the bloodstream. There is no cure for this disease; rather, it is managed over a lifetime by taking insulin, which decreases the amount of sugar in the blood. Similar to this, addiction must be managed, to ensure the substance use does not return. Therefore, the goal of treatment is not a cure but rather remission, in which the addictive behaviors and symptoms have stopped but preventive measures must still be taken to ensure there is no relapse. Relapse is the reactivation of an addiction after a period of abstinence or remission.

Treatments are generally multipronged and include one-on-one therapy or counseling sessions, group sessions such as Narcotics Anonymous where people meet to discuss and share their struggles and successes with addiction, and pharmacological therapies such as methadone or Suboxone (buprenorphine and naloxone) for opioid addiction or nicotine gums and patches for nicotine addiction. Often those who are dependent on a substance and desire to quit will begin by signing into a detox center and then attending a rehab program. Those who become addicted often face a lifetime struggle to abstain from their addictive behaviors. Even for those who have been able to overcome an addiction for a long period of time, in many cases even after years of abstaining, there is always a risk of relapse. The greatest risk of relapse comes when people encounter triggers, such as ones described above. Three triggers are known to cause the greatest risk of relapse: stress, reexposure to a drug, and environmental cues. Examples of stressful events include deaths of loved ones, increased job demands, loss of job, relationship problems, failed relationships, injury, and others. Stressful events lead to relapse due to attempts by the brain to override stressful feelings with reward feelings from the addictive substances and behaviors. Users often attempt to use a substance again "just once," but when an addictive substance is reintroduced to the body, this reexposure causes drug-priming, where the use of a drug after a period of abstinence quickly causes a heavy return in craving for the drug, thus increasing the likelihood of restarting regular use. For treatment of psychological dependence, behavioral techniques are often utilized during recovery to help decrease the triggering of conditioned, automatic behaviors a person has learned by association with environmental cues and situations.

Risk Factors in Acquiring Addiction

What determines who gets addicted and who does not get addicted? As is the case with essentially all mental health disorders, the answer is that likelihood of addiction for any one person is a combination of genetic, psychological, social, environmental, and cultural factors. Those who are never exposed to a drug cannot become addicted. Social stigma or acceptance related to substance use affects the likelihood a person will use a drug, and it also affects the lengths a person would go to in order to hide his or her addiction. Those who have less exposure to triggers will have less tendency to relapse.

Addiction runs in families, and so if one generation has struggled with addiction, it is likely the next will struggle as well. One of the reasons it seems to run in families is due to increased social acceptance and exposure to substance use within the family. However, it has also been found that there is an increased genetic risk of addiction as well, beyond what can be accounted for by socialization alone. The strongest evidence for genetic tendency toward addiction comes from studies of twins separated at birth. Twin studies are useful in that they allow scientists to unravel the question of nature versus nurture and figure out if addiction is a completely socialized phenomenon related to exposure to drugs (nurture), or if it is more a product of genetics (nature). What has been shown is that a clear genetic component exists. Identical twins have the exact same DNA and therefore the exact same genetics. Fraternal twins (nonidentical twins) do not have the same DNA and therefore do not have the exact same genetics. When looking at the identical twins that have been separated at birth, it is found that when one identical twin has an addiction problem, the other identical twin, who was raised in a different environment, will have an addiction problem 50% of the time. When looking at fraternal twins that have been separated at birth, it is found that when one fraternal twin has an addiction problem, the other fraternal twin, who was also raised in a different environment, will have an addiction problem only 25% of the time. Therefore, identical twins separated at birth were twice as likely to share addiction problems as fraternal twins separated at birth. In this way, it was shown that socialization by itself (nurture) cannot account for whether or not a person falls prey to an addiction. If socialization completely explained the tendency toward addiction, then identical twins separated at birth would be no more likely to share addiction problems than fraternal twins.

Other studies have shown the explicit mechanism by which genetics cause a person to be prone to addiction. Those with a genetic tendency toward addiction secrete four times as much dopamine in response to a drug than those without the genetic tendency. Therefore, those with genetic tendency toward addiction experience a much greater reward and much greater "high" than those without the genetic tendency. These truths about the genetics of addiction are so important to realize given the common perception that addiction is merely a choice or a matter of willpower. While it is certainly true that without exposure to a drug, one cannot become addicted, it is also true that among those who are exposed to a drug, certain people are much more likely to become addicted due to genetics.

In conclusion, addictive drugs cause chemical and structural changes to the brain that lessen a person's ability for self-control and lead to harm. It is easy to become frustrated with people who have substance use disorders because they make such seemingly bad choices, but the science of addiction shows that making bad choices is in fact a symptom of the disease related to its biochemical effects on the brain.

CHAPTER 3

"Downers": Sedatives, Sleep Aids, and Anxiolytics

Many of the most well-known and misused prescription drugs fall into a category called sedative-hypnotics. In brief, the overall effect of sedative-hypnotics is that they are *relaxing* (sedative) and *sleep-inducing* (hypnotic). Many of these drugs, such as the benzodiazepines, are also referred to as anxiolytics (anxiety-breaking) or tranquillizers for their ability to relieve anxiety (nervousness) and make a person feel tranquil. "Sedative-hypnotic" is an umbrella term that includes many different types of drugs. Sedative-hypnotics include multiple different classes and subgroups of drugs that differ by chemical structure and mechanism of action but that all share an ability to help people relax or to help them fall asleep. Some common examples of prescription sedative-hypnotics are alprazolam (Xanax), zolpidem (Ambien), and clonazepam (Klonopin). A useful broad conception of sedative-hypnotics is that they are considered "downer" drugs because they are central nervous system (CNS) depressants, meaning they slow down the rate of neural transmission in the brain. This is by contrast with "upper" drugs, the stimulants, which speed neural transmission. These are discussed in a later chapter. Opioids also have some downer, sedative properties, but they are considered separately in this text due to their different effects and mechanisms of action.

Xanax is a popular enough street drug that its pill form is often referred to in slang terminology as a "bar" or a "football." These names are presumably due to the unique shape of the pill, which looks like a large rectangular bar shape that can be broken up into four individual square doses. The simple name "xan" (pronounced "zan") is common as well. Numerous other prescription sedative-hypnotic are well known and are even mentioned regularly in pop culture. For example, the rapper Jay-Z mentions Ambien in the lyrics to his 2009 hit song "Empire State of Mind," where he advises listeners that New York is "the city never sleeps/better slip you an Ambien." Ambien also features prominently in the first episode of Judd Apatow's hit Netflix comedy series *Love*, in which lead character Mickey takes Ambien to attempt to go to sleep, only to change plans and go out for the night to a midnight church service. The Ambien use results in her feeling so disinhibited and relaxed that she walks onto the church stage. She appears to be intoxicated from the Ambien in a manner similar to as if she were drunk. She proceeds to deliver an inappropriately explicative-laden monologue about how love has ruined her life.

Like other prescription drugs of abuse, many of the properties that make sedative-hypnotics so useful to the medical profession also make them intrinsically susceptible to misuse. A saying among the medical community is that "if it sedates, it sells," meaning that in general, if drugs have relaxing properties, they have the potential to be diverted into street sales or other improper use. The mental effect a person feels when taking a sedative-hypnotic such as Xanax or Valium is somewhere in the ballpark of the mental effects one feels when drinking alcohol. Indeed, sedative-hypnotics are commonly paired with other downer substances such as alcohol or opioids to enhance the relaxing experience, despite the potentially fatal result of combining these substances. In the same way that alcohol is known to provide feelings of relaxation, disinhibition, euphoria, and sleepiness, similar properties can be found to varying degrees and combinations in the sedative-hypnotic drugs. Consider, for example, how the relaxing properties of alcohol are the origin of its use as a social lubricant. Decreased social anxiety makes people feel less afraid and more able to speak freely. It decreases the fear people feel in their minds, and in this way they become more disinhibited, meaning that to some degree they stop holding back from doing and saying what they want. Sedative-hypnotics and alcohol share fundamental similarities due to the fact that they share a common chemical mechanism in the brain and increase the release of gamma-aminobutyric acid (GABA), a type of neurotransmitter that slows and calms the nervous system, including the brain. Similar to alcohol, these drugs can carry dangerous side effects during short-term intoxication, such as impaired driving ability. Also similar to alcohol, consistent long-term use can result in the buildup of tolerance and lead to physical dependence of many of the sedative-hypnotic drugs. Therefore, for the average reader, alcohol intoxication is at least a rough starting point to get a feel for what it is like to have a sedative-hypnotic. Overdose of benzodiazepines decreases the body's respiratory drive, and so in users who overdose, their body does not sense that they are out of oxygen, the sensation of suffocation does not occur, no breath is taken, and the person can eventually die.

Some of the principal classes of prescription drugs that typically fall under the sedative-hypnotic category are as follows:

1) Benzodiazepines, such as alprazolam (Xanax) and lorazepam (Ativan)
2) Z-drugs, such as zolpidem (Ambien) or zaleplon (Sonata)
3) Barbiturates, such as amobarbital, butalbital, or phenobarbital

In addition to these three drugs classes, other various prescription drugs exist that are mostly used for other medical purposes but still have significant sedative, hypnotic, or anxiolytic properties that make them attractive for misuse. Some of these drugs include:

- The anesthetic drug Ketamine
- The antipsychotic drugs Quetiapine (Seroquel) and Promethazine
- The sedative-hypnotic drug Methaqualone (Quaalude, discontinued in the United States since 1985)

Each of these classes of medication works by a different biochemical mechanism to produce a variety of different psychoactive effects. However, as a general rule, most of the drugs mentioned in this chapter show strong action involving the neurotransmitter GABA.

BIOLOGY OF SEDATIVE-HYPNOTICS

GABA can be thought of as the yellow traffic light of the nervous system. When the brain is flooded with the chemical GABA, it knows to slow everything down. Benzodiazepines, barbiturates, Z-drugs, alcohol, and other drugs act strongly at sites in the brain called the $GABA_A$ receptors. When these drugs bind to the $GABA_A$ receptors, they increase the amount of GABA neurotransmitter released into the brain. The increased GABA tells the brain to slow down, take it easy, and not work so hard thinking about so many things. Each different benzodiazepine, barbiturate, and Z-drug interacts with the $GABA_A$ receptors differently, for example, by acting for a longer or shorter amount of time. In addition, each drug also has additional actions at a unique constellation of other receptors in the body that give each drug its individual character. However, in general, when discussing sedative-hypnotics, the primary mechanism of action causing the observed relaxation effects is increased release of GABA into the brain, which slows the brain function.

A BRIEF HISTORY OF SEDATIVE-HYPNOTICS

The first class of truly effective sedative-hypnotics to exist were the barbiturates, which came about in the early twentieth century. Barbiturates are much more rarely prescribed these days, but they were once some of the most highly prescribed and most misused drugs in the early twentieth century. These drugs are derivatives of a substance called barbituric acid, which has no medicinal value on its own but is the parent compound of the numerous chemicals developed from it. Barbituric acid was discovered in 1864 by a German chemist named Adolf von Baeyer, who supposedly named the compound for a lady he knew named Barbara. The molecule was synthesized from urea, which is found in urine, and diethyl malonate, an acidic molecule found in several fruits. Von Baeyer did not find any medical use for this compound. In 1903, two scientists at the Bayer pharmaceutical company named Emil Fischer and Joseph von Mering synthesized a chemical related to barbituric acid called barbital. They soon discovered this molecule was a drug that helped relieve anxiety and insomnia, and the barbiturate drug class was born. Numerous other barbiturates were developed over the next few decades, and the drug class was also found to be useful in multiple areas of medicine. They are an effective anesthesia before surgery, and they were the first medicine truly effective in the treatment of seizure disorders such as epilepsy.

The popularity of barbiturates greatly decreased after the discovery of benzodiazepines in the 1950s. Barbiturates carry much greater side effects than benzodiazepines, are far more addictive, and carry a very high risk of overdose death. In fact, a barbiturate called sodium thiopental, a short-acting anesthetic, is one of the drugs used in lethal injections given for the death penalty. Furthermore, barbiturates are extremely addicting and require several weeks to detox. Two of the most common barbiturates found today are phenobarbital, a seizure medication; and butalbital, which is sold as part of a headache medication, Fioricet, which is a combination medication that also contains acetaminophen (Tylenol) and caffeine.

The first benzodiazepine to be synthesized, chlordiazepoxide (Librium), was developed in 1957 by chemist Leo Sternbach while working at the Hoffmann-La Roche pharmaceutical company. Librium was discovered by accident during research into a class of molecules used to make dyes. Benzodiazepines have similar uses as barbiturates, but they are by comparison much safer and much less addicting. As such, they have largely replaced barbiturates in many ways. However, benzodiazepines do still carry numerous risks, and they are still some of the most highly abused prescription drugs that exist. As mentioned in the first chapter, benzodiazepines are currently the second most common drug type associated with drug overdose death in the United States after opioid medications.

Methaqualone (Quaalude), also known as "quaaludes," "'ludes," or "disco biscuits," is a barbiturate-like drug that was originally developed as a malaria medication but was later found to have sedative-hypnotic properties. For a time, methaqualone was commonly prescribed as a sleep aid, and it eventually gained widespread popularity in the 1960s and 1970s as a club drug. Originally marketed as having no addictive or abuse potential, and initially not even categorized as a controlled substance, these drugs were soon found to have effects similar to barbiturates and other sedative-hypnotics. They were popular for their relaxing high, and they were thought to specifically decrease sexual inhibition, a feature highly prized during the decade's sexual revolution. Toward the middle of the decade, there were increasing reports of overdoses on methaqualone, in particular when mixed with alcohol. It also gained a reputation as a date rape drug. Methaqualone was eventually recategorized as a Schedule I drug by the DEA, and it has been unavailable in the United States since 1985. Of note, it is still commonly abused in South Africa. Quaaludes' reputation as a date rape drug came back into the public discourse in 2015 when the media released a surge of reports of sexual assaults committed over many years by comedian Bill Cosby in which he regularly gave quaaludes to women in order to incapacitate them.

The Z-drugs, such as zolpidem (Ambien), zaleplon (Sonata), and zopiclone (Zimovane), are similar to benzodiazepines but interact with the GABA$_A$ receptors in a slightly different way. Zopiclone was the first be developed and was introduced in 1986. As a result, they have limited use mostly as hypnotics to help people fall asleep. They are not generally prescribed for sedative properties. Z-drugs are thought to result in a better, more natural quality of sleep than what would be gained from a benzodiazepine. Z-drugs do not alter the body's natural cycle of sleep phases, whereas benzodiazepines cause changes in the sleep phase.

Most of this chapter will be devoted to discussing benzodiazepines. Benzodiazepines play a crucial role in the treatment variety of disorders that involve intolerable anxiety, such as panic disorder, generalized anxiety disorder, or the intense anxiety patients feel after receiving a heart transplant. These drugs can be used for brief periods to help induce sleep for those suffering from insomnia. They are often used during detox from alcohol or other substances for those suffering physical withdrawal symptoms such as tremors or hallucinations. They are also the drug of choice used with epilepsy patients during active seizures, since their neuron-relaxing effects can slow down the overexcited electrical activity in the brain and break the seizure before it causes permanent brain damage or death. Benzodiazepines are much more commonly abused in today's society than the other prescription drugs in this category.

However, before going into further detail about the medical uses of benzodiazepines, it is useful to discuss in further detail one of the most common conditions that benzodiazepines and other sedatives are supposed to treat: anxiety.

THE NATURE OF ANXIETY

When benzodiazepines or other drugs are discussed in terms of their effect on a person's emotional state, they are referred to as anxiolytics.

The word "anxiolytic" comes from combining the word "anxiety" and the Greek word ending "-lysis" (breaking apart). Therefore, one of the principal uses of this drug class is that they cut through a person's anxiety.

Anxiety is one of the most basic emotional states that humans experience. Anxiety can be mild or severe. It is known by many names such as fear, terror, apprehension, worry, dread, uneasiness, nervousness, panic, and other names that denote the level and quality of anxiety that a person is feeling. Other basic emotional states people feel are sadness, anger, surprise, disgust, and happiness.

It is often helpful and healthy to experience anxiety for short periods of time. In the evolutionary sense, anxiety is considered a useful tool for survival that developed in order to alert the organism that something is dangerous. For example, if a hiker is walking in the woods and sees a snake in the path, a fear or anxiety response occurs. When anxiety and stress levels are manageable, they can serve as motivation. For example, a student might feel anxiety about failing an upcoming test, and this may motivate him or her to study and do homework in order to decrease this anxiety about failing. Some readers may have doubt that anxiety is a problem that requires any treatment at all. Many will note that anxiety is a normal emotion that all people have. However, certain people develop levels of anxiety that are far above and beyond what the average person experiences as anxiety, so high as to prevent them from performing necessary functions in life such as school, work, or maintaining stable relationships. It is this level of heightened anxiety that would require treatment. This is analogous to the body's experience of pain. All people experience mild forms of pain throughout their life that require no pain medication, such as minor scratches or abrasions. However, there are people with conditions that cause pain so severe—for example, pain from cancer that has spread into the bones—that only treatment with a strong pain medication like an opioid can work. A further analogy can be made to a condition such as high blood pressure. Every human being has blood pressure, and so to have blood pressure is completely normal. However, when a person's blood pressure is too high, this become dangerous to the body and can result in damage to the brain, heart, or other organs. Blood pressure itself is normal and necessary. High blood pressure is harmful.

It is important to note that the effects of emotional states are not merely confined to the mind. Changes in emotional states correspond with physical changes across the body. For example, when a person perceives danger, a special part of the nervous system is activated called the sympathetic nervous system. When the sympathetic nervous system is activated, a person quickly goes through numerous mental and physical changes.

For example, imagine a caveman and cavewoman walking out in the forest looking for food, when suddenly they encounter an angry bear.

Their brains receive sensory information from their eyes and ears that allows them to perceive this angry bear. Their brains know through prior learning and experience that angry bears are dangerous, and a sort of danger alarm goes off in the brain that activates the sympathetic nervous system (as well as the stress/cortisol system). This activation of the sympathetic nervous system sends signals across the whole body to prepare that person to respond to the threat. The sympathetic nervous system contains nerves stretching from the brain to the abdomen that connect the brain to the adrenal glands, which sit on top of the kidneys. In response, these glands release the hormone called adrenalin (also known as epinephrine) into the bloodstream. In response to this rush of adrenalin, the caveman and cavewoman become afraid, they become more activated and energetic, their muscles tense up, their eyes dilate wide, their concentration increases, their breathing rates increase, their heartbeats race, and their circulatory system increases the blood flow to their brains and their skeletal muscles. The reason all these changes and more have occurred to the body are that adrenalin has primed the body for "fight or flight mode." If they want to live, they have the choice of either attacking the bear and killing it before it kills them, or they can decide it is too dangerous and run away from the situation to escape death. Either way, fight or flight, the sympathetic nervous system has primed their body for action. With the extra blood flow to the brain, the mind has become sharp and attentive to its surroundings. Blood flow has increased to the muscles of the arms and legs so that these muscles can get the extra oxygen they will need for the increased activity they are about to undergo while fighting or running. The heart rate and breathing have increased to pull extra oxygen from the air to replace this extra oxygen being used by the muscles. The eyes have become wide to take in all their surroundings to perceive maximum threats. All of these physical changes to the body increase the odds that this caveman and cavewoman will live to see another day (and in evolutionary terms, live to produce greater numbers of offspring).

All of these performance-enhancing changes sound great, but they come with a price. The anxious, tense state and all the fear, dread, and worry caused by seeing the bear cause physical and emotional stress to the body. A person can only fight so many bears in one day before experiencing physical and mental exhaustion. Constant running from bears is not exactly an ideal way to live. Anxiety is a *feeling*, and compared to happiness, it doesn't *feel good.*

This exhaustion caused by an overly taxed fear response is why anxiety over the long term is so detrimental to people, and this is a large reason why anxiety medications are so important for so many people. Most people no longer live in a world where they are being attacked by bears, but our abstract society has presented us with countless bears of the metaphorical variety. Eviction notices are bears when one's finances do not feel secure. Your boss is a bear if you fear she will fire you. An airplane is a bear if you're scared to fly.

Different people respond to fear in different ways. If the cavewoman is a very skilled huntress and is able to easily kill the bear each time she encounters one, the stress response she feels upon seeing a bear will become less and less. After she has defeated dozens of vicious bears, she will likely reach an emotional state where she feels proud of her accomplishments and confident in her abilities. Happiness will become mixed in the anxiety, and she will feel less fear about the whole situation. Fighting bears may even become an enjoyable adrenaline rush to her. She will have no fear of going into the woods to find food.

By contrast, what if the caveman does not fare so well in his encounters with the bears? Perhaps he has had mostly unsuccessful hunting experiences. When he sees the bear, he calculates that he will not defeat it, and so he runs away. But perhaps he is not so great a runner either, and he is nearly mauled to death by this bear. Though he narrowly escapes, this is not a situation he would like to repeat. And yet next time he is in the woods, another bear chases him, and again he narrowly escapes, this time with a scar from a claw that almost caught him. After dozens of such near-death, traumatic experiences, the caveman will likely become so deathly afraid of bears that he even becomes fearful of the forest itself. Even the sight of the trees causes him anxiety at this point, because they likely indicate that a bear is near. His behavior becomes more inhibited, and he avoids going to the woods. He takes less risks. As a result, the anxiety is beginning to spread throughout his life. If his anxiety continues to increase and spread as time goes by, he might eventually develop a generalized anxiety disorder. If he grows concerned about how his poor hunting skills will affect his relationships with other cave people, he may develop social anxiety disorder. Even worse, given that he experienced the trauma of nearly losing his life to the bears, he might develop a post-traumatic stress disorder (PTSD). If he becomes so inhibited that he can no longer take care of himself—for example, by not being able to find food he needs in the woods—then this anxiety will have reached a level that it is having significant negative effects on his health.

This is a gross simplification of how anxiety develops, and a description of the full nature of anxiety is beyond the scope of this book. However, this has hopefully given the reader a basic idea of how anxiety can increase beyond the level of normal, healthy anxiety, to a point where it is so pervasive as to affect a person's ability to live a healthy life. This is why treatment is indicated for anxiety disorders. When anxiety is experienced at a healthy, manageable level, it helps a person achieve his or her goals. When the body develops disproportionate or misplaced anxiety, it can then become harmful or detrimental to the person. Such maladaptive states are called anxiety disorders. For example, there are some people whose brains are unable to shut off the anxiety response, and thus they live in a perpetual state of anxiety (stress, worry, terror, nervousness, etc.) called generalized anxiety disorder in which excessive worries about nearly all aspects of life develop, and the person cannot relax because he or she lives in constant fear that catastrophe could strike at any moment. The fear is so great that it causes impairment in their relationships, school, work, or other important area of life. Which can be quite detrimental to their health. Another example of an anxiety disorder is panic disorder. In this disorder, a person develops intense episodes of fear and panic lasting minutes to hours in which they experience intense fear of impending doom, death, or fear they are "going crazy." During these episodes, they may experience increased heart rate, chest pain, shortness of breath, dizziness, sweating, nausea, or other sensations.

BENZODIAZEPINES

Benzodiazepines, also commonly known as "benzos," currently have the widest applicability of any sedative-hypnotics, and they have been used through the years for many functions including acute anxiety, insomnia, muscles spasms, seizures, certain withdrawal syndromes, restless leg syndromes, and even as sedation for agitated psychotic patients when they are out of touch with reality and at risk of harming themselves or others. The first benzodiazepine, chlordiazepoxide (Librium) was discovered in 1955, and this drug was first commercially available in 1960. Benzodiazepines quickly gained popularity. In 1977, they were the most prescribed class of medications in the world. It used to be thought that benzodiazepines were nonaddictive, but time has proven this to be incorrect. As a result, the prescription of benzodiazepines has dropped in recent years as doctors have become more aware of their potential dangers. Anxiety has become more often treated with antidepressant medications such as fluoxetine (Prozac), and insomnia has become more often treated with Z-drugs. Nonetheless, prescription of benzodiazepines remains common. Commonly used benzodiazepines are alprazolam (Xanax), clonazepam (Klonopin), lorazepam (Ativan), diazepam (Valium), and midazolam (Versed).

Benzodiazepines have been used historically for a multitude of anxiety disorders, such as generalized anxiety disorder, panic disorder, or specific phobias, although today they are not generally the first-line choice to treat any of these disorders, in part because of their addictive potential. Benzodiazepines are powerful drugs with strong effects that take place relatively quickly, often within 30 minutes. Assuming the dose is adequate, benzodiazepines work essentially 100% of the time, and they can take effect within 30 minutes, as opposed to a month with antidepressants. The ability to help people relax quickly is key to understanding the appeal of benzodiazepines for both medical and nonmedical uses. Anxiety, worry, stress, and other similar emotions can be very uncomfortable, even painful emotions to experience, and these drugs help to erase those feelings for a period of time. This can potentially be very useful in the short term in a condition such as panic disorder, where the distress of the panic episode is so severe, and a Xanax can help this feeling go away.

Benzodiazepines can become problematic, however, when a person starts to rely on the benzodiazepine to make her feel better whenever she is anxious, and so a habit forms in which a person learns to take a benzo, which can be dangerous. Furthermore, the longer a patient stays on the benzo, the more he gains tolerance to the drug and increases his physical dependence. For these and other reasons, the current treatment of choice for most anxiety disorders are actually the antidepressant medications— for example, Prozac (fluoxetine), Zoloft (sertraline), or Paxil (paroxetine), which have no addictive quality. Studies and clinical experience have shown that antidepressant drugs are equally as useful for the treatment of anxiety as they are for the treatment of depression.

A major drawback to the antidepressant medications in comparison to benzodiazepines is that antidepressants take much longer to have an effect. Whereas benzodiazepines work generally within 30 minutes to an hour, patients taking antidepressants should expect to take the medications for two to four weeks before they begin to feel any effect. For this reason, benzodiazepines can be useful for some patients for a short time during the initial treatment stages of disorders such as generalized anxiety disorder or major depressive disorder (major depression is often accompanied with anxiety symptoms). During the initial weeks of treatment, when the patient is just starting the antidepressant medications, benzodiazepines can be used as a "bridge" to provide quick relief to the anxiety for a few weeks until the antidepressants start to take effect.

Another common example of when a doctor might prescribe a benzodiazepine is to give a one-time dose to people with a specific phobia. A common phobia requiring treatment with a benzodiazepine is the claustrophobia a patient feels when getting imaging in an MRI (magnetic resonance imaging) machine. MRIs are important diagnostic machines that produce highly detailed images of the body's internal structures, and they are commonly used to identify evidence of disease inside a person's body. Images produced by an MRI frequently help doctors save patients' lives by identifying different types of cancers, internal infections and abscesses, autoimmune diseases such as multiple sclerosis, and others. Despite the MRI machine's good reputation for diagnosing disease and for saving lives, many patients cannot tolerate the imaging procedure due to its requiring them to be in a small enclosed area for a lengthy period of time. A typical MRI machine looks like a very large and heavy white cube, taller than the average person. In the middle of the cube is a narrow tube not much wider in diameter than the width of a person's body. Out from this narrow tube comes a flat platform on which the patient must lie down. Once the patient has lay down, the platform retracts back into the machine and pulls the patient into the narrow tunnel. Once in the tunnel, depending on where on the body the imaging will take place, the patient's motion may be highly constricted—for example, not being able to sit all the way up. Patients can often be in the tunnel for 45 minutes. During the procedure, they wear earplugs because the machine continually makes loud, grating noises, almost as bad as fingernails scraping across a chalkboard. This situation of being temporarily trapped in a loud, buzzing machine can feel intolerable to many patients. Thus, most physicians would prescribe a one-time dose of a benzodiazepine such as lorazepam (Ativan) to a claustrophobic patient before the MRI starts so that she could tolerate the procedure. Similarly, many patients who need life-saving surgeries may still feel incredibly anxious and frightened about getting the surgery. A benzodiazepine could become useful to offer patients before a surgical procedure to help them manage their anxiety. Midazolam is commonly prescribed by dentists for dental phobia (fear of dental treatment), and it is also used for patients on life-supporting mechanical ventilators to help them relax and feel more comfortable.

In addition to anxiety disorders, benzodiazepines can be life-saving in the treatment of seizure disorders such as epilepsy. Seizures are potentially life-threatening events caused by abnormally increased electrical impulses in the brain, often leading to convulsions and loss of consciousness. Due to their ability to slow the activity of the nervous system, benzodiazepines have powerful anticonvulsant properties. If a patient is found to be convulsing and having a seizure, a STAT order is placed to inject the patient with a benzodiazepine in order to stop the seizure before it becomes dangerous. Some patients require multiple injections. During a classic generalized, full-body, "tonic-clonic" seizure, a person is at increased risk from fall-related injuries (from sudden loss of consciousness) or from inhaling their own vomit. If a seizure persists for longer than five minutes, permanent damage to the nervous system, including the brain, can occur. Benzodiazepines such as lorazepam (Ativan) or midazolam (Versed) are frequently used. Clonazepam (Klonopin) can be used on a regular, daily basis to prevent seizures in Lennox-Gastaut syndrome, a rare disorder in which patients have severe recurrent and frequent seizures.

Benzodiazepines are also frequently used in the treatment of psychiatric patients who become acutely agitated and aggressive—for example, due to mania or psychosis. The long-term treatment for these brain states involves antipsychotic and mood-stabilizing medications, but in the short term, until the psychosis and mania resolve, patients may need sedation from a benzodiazepine if they appear to be an immediate danger to themselves or others. Psychosis and mania are brain states often seen in patients who suffer from psychiatric disorders such as bipolar disorder, schizoaffective disorder, or schizophrenia. Psychosis and mania may also be induced by intoxication with certain drugs. In psychotic brain states, patients lose the ability to understand what is real and what is not real. The psychosis brain state is one in which a person experiences delusions, hallucinations, and disorganized thoughts. Psychotic delusions are often of a paranoid nature—for example, feeling strongly that thoughts are being beamed into one's head by satellites or a computer chip has been planted into one's body. Hallucinations in psychosis often take the form of hearing voices that are not there. Disorganized thoughts in psychosis are evidenced by disorganized speech, such as the "word salad" phenomenon where the psychotic person's sentence structure may be composed of words and ideas that are completely disconnected from each other and make no coherent sense. Given the proper antipsychotic medications, these delusions, hallucinations, and thoughts may dissipate for a time. Mania, seen in bipolar disorder and schizoaffective disorder, is a state of elevated mood that can last for days to weeks. In a way, it can be viewed as almost the opposite of depression. In a classical, textbook representation of mania, the patient becomes extremely energetic, has a consistently and inappropriately elevated mood (can be an extremely happy and euphoric mood or an extremely angry mood), does not require sleep for several days (despite the lack of sleep, does not feel fatigued the next day as in insomnia), has increased goal-directed activity, has delusions of grandeur (e.g., thinking he or she is literally God), has free-flowing and highly rapid speech that cannot be interrupted ("pressured speech"), and engages in highly disinhibited, risky behavior such as spending all their money, spontaneously driving across the country on a "mission from God," or engaging in indiscriminate sex with multiple partners. Manic patients often have additional psychotic symptoms on top of the manic symptoms. States of drug-induced mania or drug-induced psychosis can be induced from certain illicit drugs—for example, PCP ("angel dust"), cathinone derivatives (bath salts), or synthetic cannabinoids ("K2," "spice," or "mojo").

Patients who fall into states of mania and psychosis may become so violent, paranoid, aggressive, delusional, hallucinatory, and out of touch with reality that they sometimes are brought to the emergency room by police or family for psychiatric evaluation and treatment. In a medical setting like the emergency room or an inpatient psychiatric hospital, if there is concern that a patient poses an imminent threat to himself or others, benzodiazepines are often used to calm him down before anyone can be hurt. For example, a paranoid psychotic patient may believe that the other patients around him and the nursing staff are all really demons plotting to kill him. The danger this patient feels may then put him in fight or flight mode and cause him to act in "self-defense" if he feels the demons about to attack him. Psychiatric staff can try many verbal techniques to convince these patients to take an oral, pill form of a benzodiazepine such as Ativan to help calm them down. If they cannot be calmed down or convinced to take medication orally, and they continue to engage in threatening behaviors, they might have to be manually restrained by security guards and then given an intramuscular injection of a benzodiazepine such as lorazepam (Ativan) combined with an antipsychotic medication such as haloperidol. The purpose of sedating mentally ill patients against their will during emergency situations is to decrease any immediate danger so that they can receive proper treatment to restore their ability be in touch with reality.

Before moving away from this subject, it is important to note that although states of mania and psychosis can cause patients with mental illness to become violent, it is much more often the case that mentally ill patients are the victims of violence. Patients with schizophrenia, schizoaffective disorder, and bipolar disorder often have considerable difficulty navigating everyday life, especially in times when they are not able to distinguish well what is real and what is not real. Many patients with mental illness end up homeless due to their disease, and it is more often the case that these patients are the victims or robbery or violence, rather than the perpetrators of it.

DANGERS OF BENZODIAZEPINE ABUSE

Benzodiazepines have the advantage of being generally highly effective, but they also have undesirable side effects that make them dangerous in abuse. These side effects include sedation and grogginess, confusion, decreased respiratory drive, decreased balance leading to falls, and physiologic dependence. Withdrawal from benzodiazepines is potentially fatal in that it can cause seizures. As was stated in the first chapter, benzodiazepines are the second-highest cause of prescription drug overdose deaths in the United States after opioids. In 2015, there were a total of 9,000 benzodiazepine-related drug overdose deaths in the United States.

Motives for abusing benzodiazepines differ. Some take the medications to feel high, but it appears that self-treatment of anxiety and self-treatment of insomnia are some of the key motivators that lead people to misuse benzodiazepines. These drugs are particularly appealing to those with poor coping strategies or poor tolerance to uncomfortable emotions. Given what was previously described about the nature of anxiety, it becomes easier to see how anxiety, particularly anxiety caused by trauma, could be such a burden on a patient that she would seek self-treatment in the form of benzodiazepines.

Benzodiazepines are not usually a cause of overdose on their own, but the problem occurs when they are mixed with other substances. Most often, these deaths occur from mixing benzodiazepines with substances like alcohol or opioids. Benzodiazepine overdose death occurs due to the drugs' ability to cause respiratory depression, which is a decrease in the body's drive to breathe. Breathing is both a voluntary and involuntary action. Humans have the ability to take voluntary, conscious control of their breathing if they so choose. However, most of the time, we do not take conscious control of our breathing. Receptors in the brain and circulatory system have carbon dioxide receptors that measure how much carbon dioxide is in the blood, and when this carbon dioxide reaches a certain high level, the brain causes a breath to take place. If a person chooses not to breathe, they experience what is known as dyspnea, which is the uncomfortable feeling one gets when one doesn't breathe for a long enough time. This is how we are able to remain breathing even when we are asleep. Someone who is on a high enough dose of benzodiazepine, especially when paired with other drugs that reduce the respiratory drive such as alcohol or opiates, will not feel the urge to breathe, will not have any feeling of suffocation, and will die of lack of oxygen.

Daily users of benzodiazepines can develop tolerance to the drugs and become at risk for withdrawal syndromes. Some patients become tolerant through illegal use of benzodiazepines, while other become tolerant due to long-term prescription of these medications by their physician. Currently, benzodiazepines are only advised to be prescribed for short-term treatment of anxiety and insomnia, generally for two to four weeks at a time. However, often their use is prescribed for much longer periods of time, and then the patient develops physiologic dependence. When benzos were first developed, it was thought that they were not addictive. Clinical experience over the decades has shown that this is not the case. Benzodiazepines have lower addictive potential than barbiturates, yet they do show a tendency to become addictive. In animal studies, mice have been shown to prefer places where benzodiazepines were found, and they will learn to press a lever that dispenses benzodiazepines.

Benzodiazepines may cause both short- and long-term cognitive and psychiatric problems. Daily users may experience a feeling of cognitive "cloudiness." Studies have shown that short- and long-term users of benzodiazepines will have decreased concentration. Learning and the formation of new memories are affected in that users will have increased difficulty retaining facts (procedural memory such as how to perform a physical task is not affected except possible with lorazepam). Elderly patients with dementia are particularly prone to decreased cognitive ability from benzodiazepine use as they can easily become delirious. In addition to the cognitive cloudiness experienced by daily users of benzodiazepines, there is some evidence that benzodiazepine users may be at increased risk of getting Alzheimer's disease.

The risk of accident and injury is greatly increased in benzodiazepine intoxication. Reaction time, such as a driver's time to react to an obstacle on the road, is decreased. These medications tend to decrease coordination and cause balance problems, so the elderly are particularly prone to increased falls and hip fractures with use of benzodiazepines. Elderly patients tend to use multiple prescription medications for disorders such as hypertension (increased blood pressure) or heart problems. The more medications that are added to a person's regimen, the greater the risk of drug-drug interactions and side effects such as drops in blood pressure and lightheadedness.

Alcoholics should take particular care with benzodiazepines as many of these drugs are metabolized by the liver, and thus patients with cirrhosis may metabolize these drugs quite slowly. This causes the benzodiazepines to build up in the blood to high concentrations, multiplying their side effects and increasing the potential for overdose death.

One member of the benzodiazepine family has a particularly bad and dangerous reputation as perhaps the most well-known date rape drug. This is the drug called flunitrazepam (Rohypnol), better known as "ruffies" or "roofies" in the common usage. Flunitrazepam is tasteless and odorless, and its abuse potential involves a perpetrator sneaking the drug into a victim's drink and causing this person to become sedated, leaving the victim unable to resist a sexual assault. What makes Rohypnol particularly dangerous is that in addition to producing a sedating effect, it causes "anterograde amnesia," which means that in addition to becoming sedated, the drug victim will not remember what occurred during the time the drug is in effect.

Benzodiazepine Tolerance and Withdrawal

Benzodiazepines can give a feeling of euphoria. Any drug that can give a feeling of euphoria has potential to be addicting. Once addiction forms, tolerance can form.

When the body builds tolerance and becomes physically dependent on benzodiazepines, this can lead to benzodiazepine withdrawal if the medication is stopped abruptly. Withdrawal from benzodiazepines and other sedative-hypnotics can be life-threatening in that patients can develop seizures. Conceptually, symptoms of benzodiazepine withdrawal can be thought of as the opposite of the effect that benzodiazepines have on the body. These withdrawal symptoms include rebound anxiety, panic attacks, rebound insomnia, tremors, sweating, elevated blood pressure, elevated heart rate, dilated pupils, confusion and cognitive problems, headaches, auditory hallucinations (hearing voices), visual hallucinations (such as colored lights), mania, and psychosis. Symptoms of benzodiazepine withdrawal can begin hours after cessation of benzodiazepine use, and can last up to 14 days. Benzodiazepines are also the treatment of choice for treatment of alcohol withdrawal syndrome and barbiturate withdrawal syndrome, both of which have similar symptoms to benzodiazepine withdrawal, as well as barbiturate withdrawal. To prevent these potentially deadly withdrawal syndromes, a slowly decreasing, tapered dosing of benzodiazepines given over multiple days is required to wean patients off these medications. This type of planned, controlled weaning of a patient off a substance they have dependence on is called detoxification, or detox as it is commonly known.

Benzodiazepines can be detected in the urine for up to three days for occasional users or between four and six weeks for those who have used regularly for over a year. They can be detected for up to 90 days in the hair. They can be detected in the blood for between 6 and 48 hours. False positives can occur in people who take the antidepressant medication sertraline (Zoloft) or the arthritis drug oxaprozin.

OTHER COMMONLY ABUSED SEDATING DRUGS

Beyond the sedative-hypnotics, there are numerous other prescription drugs with sedating properties that are regularly abused. Certain tricyclic antidepressants are sedating, such as amitriptyline. These drugs are sometimes useful in treating chronic pain syndromes. Heroin users will frequently use amitriptyline to augment their high, which is dangerous due to amitriptyline's numerous side effects including erratic heart rhythms. Opiates themselves have sedative qualities, although this is generally not their primary use. The antipsychotic medication promethazine has sedating effects and was a popular drug of abuse in the 1990s hip-hop scene in the form of "purple drank." Also known as "sizzurp," purple drank is a concoction of Sprite or Mountain Dew mixed with prescription-strength cough syrup containing the opioid drug codeine and promethazine. When drunk with alcohol, it can cause respiratory depression leading to overdose. The muscle relaxant Flexeril also has some sedating and mildly euphoric properties, giving it abuse potential. It works on a subtype of GABA receptors called $GABA_B$ receptors.

KETAMINE: MEDICAL USES

Ketamine is a prescription drug with unique properties that is sometimes grouped with the sedatives. It was developed in 1962 as a form of anesthesia by Parke-Davis laboratories. Ketamine is a derivative of the illicit drug phencyclidine, or PCP (also known as "angel dust," "peace," or other terms), and it has gained status in recent years as a potent "club drug," and its misuse is widespread across many countries. It has distinct dissociative and psychedelic effects not seen in other sedative-hypnotics. Its effects can range from mild relaxation and euphoria at low doses to dissociative "out-of-body" experiences at higher doses.

Medically, ketamine is most often used as a form of anesthesia, particularly in emergency situations. Unlike many other forms of anesthesia, ketamine does not cause drops in blood pressure, so it is useful in combat zones or other trauma situations where patients may have low blood pressure due to blood loss or other causes.

Interest in the use of ketamine by psychiatrists to treat depression has increased in recent years as well. Although its use for this purpose is still not widespread, there has been some evidence that periodic infusions of ketamine may be effective in patients for whom other depression treatments have been ineffective.

Even more so than in human medicine, ketamine is often used as an anesthetic in veterinary medicine. In particular, it is used to sedate large, uncooperative animals at a distance.

Ketamine is primarily an NMDA receptor blocker, blocking the effects of the neurotransmitter called glutamate. It also has some action at the opioid receptors, giving it analgesic (pain-relieving) properties. It also appears to activate sedating GABA receptors as well as euphoria-inducing dopamine receptors.

RECREATIONAL USE OF KETAMINE

Ketamine usually is packaged in vials of liquid called ampules, but it is commonly used by drying it out to form a powder or crystals, which are then snorted or ingested. Injection is also possible. Ketamine was first used recreationally in the 1970s among medical and veterinary professionals, and its popularity has continued to grow. In the 1990s, it became associated with the gay dance scene in the United Kingdom. Ketamine's effects differ greatly at smaller doses as compared to larger doses, and today it continues to be used primarily in dance and rave scenes all over the world. It is frequently used in home environments, where users feel safe and comfortable.

Ketamine's effects last about two to three hours. Due to its unique chemical properties, it has distinct effects at lower doses than it does at higher doses. At lower doses, ketamine acts largely as a stimulant, providing increased energy, focus, a "trippy" feeling, and feeling of well-being (euphoria). At higher doses, more dissociative, psychedelic, and sedating effects predominate. Users will sometimes take ketamine at doses high enough that they experience a unique state of consciousness called a "K-hole" in slang terminology. Users have described this K-hole state of consciousness as feeling almost completely dissociated from or "outside of" themselves, unaware of their identity or existence, and experiencing a state where they feel they are traveling through a dark tunnel into light. Coming out of the trip, they may at first know their name, realize they have a body, or know they are human.

DANGERS OF KETAMINE

Ketamine use often include periods of amnesia, and users may lose track of how much they are using because they may forget they recently took another dose. Due to its anesthetic properties, users also have decreased ability to feel pain. As a result, they can sustain injuries that they do not recognize until the drug has worn off. They may become the victim of sexual abuse and not feel or remember it. At high enough doses, ketamine produces a psychotic state nearly identical to that exhibited by patients with schizophrenia. Ketamine users can therefore experience delusions, auditory and visual hallucinations, disconnected thoughts, decreased cognitive ability, and bizarre behavior. Indeed, ketamine is sometimes used by research scientists to induce a schizophrenia-like state in order to research the disease. Users can sometimes find themselves admitted to psychiatric hospitals for psychosis. Ketamine is less dangerous in overdose than many of the sedative-hypnotics such as benzodiazepines.

CHAPTER 4

"Painkillers": Opioids and Opiates

Despite the opioid crisis taking hold of the nation, opioid medications are indispensable in medical care, and they are unlikely to go away anytime soon. Some of the most highly recognizable medications are opioids, such as oxycodone-acetaminophen (Percocet) or hydromorphone (Vicodin). There is no other class of medications on earth that can match the analgesic (pain-relieving) qualities of opioid medications. There are numerous medical conditions—for example, cancers that metastasize (spread) to the bone—in which the resulting pain is so unbearable that no pain medication other than opioids can touch it. The cancer eats away at their bodies. Metastasis may occur in their vertebrae, their hip bones, their brains, their livers, and other places in the body. Cancers can fill the lungs and make it highly uncomfortable and difficult to breathe. There is not a cure to treat every illness. In hospice centers across the world, there are countless patients who have terminal illnesses, unbearable pain, and no hope for cure. These are patients who have a life expectancy of less than six months. If it were not for opioids, patients with many incurable diseases would die long, excruciating deaths. Opioids are crucial in treating pain after many types of surgery.

Opioids are some of the most powerful medications that exist, and through history they have proved to be both a blessing and a curse to humanity. Opioids have numerous beneficial and pleasurable effects that make them susceptible to abuse. Additionally, they have numerous dangerous side effects that make them dangerous when misused. In addition to relieving pain, many opioids produce a "high" feeling of euphoria by directly stimulating the mesolimbic dopamine pathway. Opioids have some anxiolytic and sedative (CNS depressant) properties, making them relaxing to take. All too often, however, these soothing effects act like a siren's call, lulling the user into a false sense of well-being and resulting in an overdose. The renowned musician and songwriter Prince, who wrote such classic songs as "Purple Rain" and "When Doves Cry," was found to have died from fentanyl overdose, according to his autopsy report. Another famous musician and songwriter who died recently, Tom Petty, was found to have multiple prescription drugs, including benzodiazepines and opiates, in his system. Drugs found in his toxicology report included fentanyl, oxycodone, temazepam, alprazolam, acetylfentanyl, and despropionyl fentanyl.

This chapter will focus less on the epidemiology of the opioid crisis and more on the actual effects of the drugs themselves on individuals in terms of their medical uses as well as their potential for harm. This chapter will also discuss the differences among the multitude of opioid medications that exist. More about the possible causes of the opioid epidemic will be discussed in later chapters.

BIOLOGY OF OPIOIDS

Perhaps the greatest reason that opioid medications are so effective is that human bodies are designed to have opioids relieve their pain. In fact, just as there are multiple types of opioid medications, our own bodies produce their own multitude of opioids, called endogenous opioids. The most famous of these are called endorphins. These endorphin molecules are famous for giving runners a "runner's high." Endorphins operate at the exact same receptors as opioid drugs, and they have many of the same effects, such as pain relief and euphoria. The word "endorphin" came from combining the words "endogenous" and "morphine." The word endogenous indicates that something was made within the body, so the word endorphin literally means "morphine produced within the body."

The runner's high is a useful example of how the body uses endorphins. When the muscles are stressed during vigorous running, they become slightly torn and broken down in the process. Ultimately, this slight breaking down of muscle tissue is a positive process for the runner since this manageable amount of stress lets the body know it's time to increase muscle buildup. Genes are activated that tell the muscle cells to increase the assembly of proteins and other molecules into larger muscle fibers to better prepare for the next run. In the meantime, until the new muscles are built up, the runner's muscles become sore from all the exertion and microscopic damage. The body responds to decrease this pain by releasing pain-relieving endorphins. The endorphins released during this activity also can give a feeling of euphoria to the runner, thereby giving a reward feeling for completing that activity. (The reward feeling, euphoria, given to a runner by endorphins is the result of chemical stimulation of the same common dopamine reward pathway that was discussed in Chapter 2. In fact, any feeling of reward or euphoria, drug based or not, ultimately is the result of this pathway. The body essentially wants to reward the person for exercising.) Thus, the very system by which the body regulates pain involves opioid molecules.

Opioid receptors were discovered in the 1960s and 1970s, and scientists discovered that the body contains multiple types of opioid receptors. These receptors, found on the surfaces of cell membranes, exist in numerous different tissues and organs throughout the body. They are mainly associated with nerve tissue and have effects on the human nervous system. For example, when a patient undergoes surgery, the scalpel's cutting of the skin activates the free nerve endings of the peripheral nervous system to send pain signals to the brain. However, if there are increased amounts of opioid medications in the body, they activate opioid receptors in the nervous system, and the pain signal is stopped from reaching the brain.

There are three main subtypes of opioid receptors with which medicine is most concerned. These subtypes are named after Greek letters and are called the *mu*, *delta*, and *kappa* receptors. Some subtypes are more commonly found in one part of the body than another. For example, the delta receptors are found in the brain only, whereas the kappa receptors are found in the brain, the spinal cord, and the peripheral nervous system as well. The mu receptors are found in the brain, spinal cord, peripheral nervous system, and also in the intestines.

Each subtype of opioid receptor produces different effects on the body when they are activated. Activated mu receptors provide pain relief and euphoria (via the dopamine common reward pathway), but they also work to increase physical dependence, cause the pupils to constrict and become small, cause the digestive tract to slow down, and cause a decrease in the respiratory drive. Thus, some of the undesirable side effects of opioids are already becoming apparent in the actions of these receptors. For example, when the digestive tract slows down, constipation occurs. When the respiratory drive decreases, a person no longer feels the uncomfortable feeling of suffocation, because his brain does not tell him he needs to breathe. Small, "pinpoint" pupils are a common sign of opioid overdose utilized by medical workers to identify opioid overdose when they find a person unconscious and don't know the reason. The delta opioid receptors also provide pain relief and may have antidepressant effects. One of the negative effects of activated delta receptors is that they also mediate physical dependence, which can also increase the likelihood a person has a seizure. The kappa opioid receptors provide pain relief, sedation, and actually protect against seizures. On the other hand, these receptors can cause depression, dissociative effects, hallucinogenic effects, stress, pinpoint pupils, and increased urination.

A BRIEF HISTORY OF OPIOIDS

Opioids get their name from opium, which is made from the dried sap, or "latex," of the flowering plant called *papaver somniferum*. This plant is commonly known as the opium poppy, and it is the same plant species used for poppy seeds, an ingredient often used in baked goods such as muffins. The opium poppy contains numerous naturally occurring molecules called opium alkaloids. The opium alkaloids are a group of similarly shaped molecules found in the opium poppy that are either directly useful as pharmaceuticals or are useful as chemical precursors for other medicines. These opium alkaloids can be found within the raw opium and also within other parts of the plant such as the stem. For example, approximately 12% of raw opium is pure morphine. Morphine is still one of the most frequently used medications today for moderate to severe pain. Some other examples of opium alkaloids found in the opium poppy are codeine, oripavine, and thebaine. Codeine is used for mild to moderate pain and also to suppress coughs in cough syrup. Oripavine and thebaine are not directly used in medicine, but they are intermediate molecules that can be converted to a variety of medicines such as oxycodone, found in extended-release form as OxyContin, or naloxone, the opioid antidote also known as Narcan.

Raw opium has been used since prehistoric times for many of the same purposes that opioids are used for today, such as pain relief, and it was used in regions of Greece, Egypt, Persia, Afghanistan, and India. The traditional method of collecting opium is still in widespread use today, especially in illegal opioid production. At the top of the stem of each opium plant is a round green seedpod about the size and shape of a chicken egg. When opium poppies bloom, these egg-shaped seedpods open to reveal large beautiful flowers, usually red, purple, or white. The opium cultivator does not wait for the plant to bloom, and instead is more interested in the seedpod. The seedpods contain a sticky liquid called opium latex, and when this latex is dried out, what's left is the raw opium. Traditional cultivators collect this opium latex by taking a knife into the field and cutting one or more slits into the side of each seedpod. Droplets of opium latex seep out from the slits, and the latex is then allowed to dry in the sun for later collection. The dried latex has a gummy texture that can then be shaped into blocks. These blocks of dried opium latex are what is referred to as "raw opium," or simply "opium."

In illegal opium production today, this opium latex is then quickly chemically converted to pure morphine base. The morphine, in turn, is then quickly converted to heroin, which is a similar molecule to morphine but has two to three times the potency, and thus is more efficient to ship. The relatively easy conversion of opium to the much more potent and compact substance heroin is one of the greatest reasons for its popularity as an illegal, black market drug.

Opium was used throughout the Middle Ages as a treatment for pain, nervousness, and sleep induction. Following the fall of the Roman Empire, its use was primarily limited to the Muslim world until the time of the Crusades, when soldiers brought opium use back to Europe. A popular form of opium at that time was a tincture of opium mixed with ethanol, called "laudanum" due to its having "laudable," praiseworthy qualities.

Due to increased global trade following the voyages of Columbus and other explorers, opium use for recreational purposes began to spread across multiple parts of the world around 1500 CE, especially in Europe, Turkey, the Middle East, and China. This recreational use accelerated through the early 1900s when it was eventually replaced globally by recreational heroin use. Recreational smoking of opium has a particularly rich history in China, once famous for "opium dens" where men would gather to smoke opium together. The practice was so widespread that the ruling emperors attempted to ban its sale multiple times unsuccessfully during these centuries. The ban on the British opium trade in China in the early 1800s was such a point of contention as to result in two "Opium Wars" between the Chinese and the British.

Medically, opium was used more or less in its raw form until the late 1800s. Its raw form was used widely even in the American Civil War by surgeons repairing battle wounds. Toward the end of the century, after syringes came into wide use, raw forms of opium began to be replaced by the more purified opioids used today.

The first purified opium alkaloid was extracted in Germany in 1807 by chemist Friedrich Serturner, and he named this drug "morphium" after the Greek god of dreams, Morpheus, due to the drug's sleep-inducing qualities. Commercial production of this drug began in 1827 by a company that eventually became the modern pharmaceutical company Merck. Morphine is still one of the most commonly used medicines for pain control even today. Since the advent of purified morphine extraction from opium, numerous other natural and synthetic products have been derived from the opium poppy.

In the late 1800s and earlier 1900s, numerous synthetic and semisynthetic opioid drugs were discovered in laboratories by altering the chemical structures of the naturally occurring opium alkaloids. These synthetic and semisynthetic opioids were initially designed to be useful as prescription drugs, but many have unfortunately also become new forms of recreational opioid used across the United States and Europe. It may surprise many people to know that heroin was initially sold by the Bayer pharmaceutical company as an over-the-counter "nonaddictive" alternative to morphine. Also known by its scientific name diamorphine, heroin was first synthesized in 1874 by C. R. Alder Wright, an English chemist working at a medical school in London. Diamorphine was first produced commercially for public consumption by the Bayer Company (makers of Bayer aspirin). Diamorphine gained the name "heroin" from the Bayer Company as part of its marketing campaign to denote its "heroic" qualities. It may also surprise readers in the United States that heroin, prescribed under the diamorphine name, is still legally prescribed in many countries. For example, it is used in the United Kingdom in pain treatment for terminally ill cancer patients. In the Netherlands, it can be prescribed to people addicted to heroin who have failed methadone treatment. In the United States, heroin is a Schedule I drug and not considered to have any medical value.

Today, the legal production of opium poppies for pharmaceutical use is tightly controlled. These plants can only be grown legally in certain spots in India, Turkey, and Australia (Tasmania), and the opium collected from them can be shipped only to a certain handful of pharmaceutical companies with the rights to make opioid medications. Most opium grown for illegal purposes is produced in four areas of the world, two in Asia and two in the Americas. In Asia, the primary locations for opium production are called the Golden Crescent and the Golden Triangle. The Golden Crescent consists of areas in Afghanistan, Iran, Pakistan. The Golden Triangle consists of mountainous regions in neighboring Myanmar, Laos, and Thailand. In the Americas, heroin is primarily produced in Mexico and Colombia. Afghanistan is by far the largest nonpharmaceutical producer of opium, producing approximately 90% of the world's supply. (Of note, Afghanistan also produces most of the world's cannabis, in the form of hashish.)

TYPES OF OPIOID MEDICATIONS

There are multiple different prescription opioid medications that exist. The major differences in the effects of these drugs are their strength, the speed at which their effects are felt, and the length of time they stay in the body. They can also differ in their side effects and routes of administration, as some are available in pill form while others are only intravenous medications.

As was noted in the previous section, numerous derivatives of the natural opium alkaloids have been developed in laboratories. As a result, one useful way to categorize opioid medications is by whether they were derived from natural sources or by using laboratory techniques. Classifying opioids in this way, the three major categories are the naturally occurring opiates, the semisynthetic opioids, and the synthetic opioids.

Naturally Occurring Opiates

The two most common naturally occurring opiate medications are morphine and codeine.

Morphine, the first pure opioid alkaloid extracted from raw opium, has remained in widespread use by medical practitioners ever since it was first discovered. Morphine is generally the first opioid medication a physician will consider to treat moderate to severe pain. This is mainly because it is relatively inexpensive and because physicians are comfortable with it, since it has been used for a very long time. Morphine is frequently used during heart attacks or during labor and delivery.

Due to its historical prominence, the pain relief given by morphine is the standard against which all other pain medications are compared. As a result, all pain medications are described in terms of how effective they are relative to morphine. For example, raw opium, which physicians used before the modern era, has only about one-tenth, or 10%, the pain-relieving strength of morphine pills. Morphine has certain drawbacks, however, that mean it will not be the best choice for all patients. For example, because morphine is mostly excreted from the body through the kidneys and into the urine, it is not the best drug to use in patients who have kidney problems, because it can stay in the blood and potentially lead to overdose.

Morphine injected into the vein is about three times as strong as morphine in pill form, because injecting the drug into the vein directly instead of swallowing it allows the drug to bypass the digestive tract including the liver, which metabolizes a significant amount of oral morphine before it reaches the blood. This principle, that the injection of drugs often results in much higher potency because it bypasses the digestive tract, is the reason that people who misuse opioids often progress to injecting them into the vein.

Codeine, another naturally occurring opiate that can be extracted from the opium poppy, has about a third of the strength of morphine, and it is used for mild to moderate pain only. Codeine is also often found in cough syrups and used as a cough suppressant.

Semisynthetic Opioids

Semisynthetic opioids are drugs that have been developed over the years by organic chemists. These chemists have invented new opioid molecules by taking naturally occurring opium alkaloids and using chemical reactions to slightly alter the shapes of the naturally occurring molecules by adding extra atoms called "functional groups." Since a molecule's properties are determined by its shape, organic chemists were able to create new semisynthetic molecules with slightly different shapes from their natural counterparts. Some of these new semisynthetic molecules, it turned out, were even better fits for the opioid receptors than even the naturally occurring opioids. In this way, scientists discovered opioid molecules that were even more potent than the naturally occurring opioids. For example, the street drug heroin is also a semisynthetic opioid. C. R. Alder Wright created heroin by essentially performing a chemical reaction of morphine with another chemical called acetic anhydride. By boiling the two chemicals together, two groups of atoms called "acetyl groups" (each made of an additional carbon atom, two oxygen atoms, and a hydrogen atom) were added to the morphine molecule, forming a new molecule with a slightly different shape from morphine. This new molecule was an even better fit into the opioid receptors and therefore more potent than the naturally occurring morphine. A new drug was born. Some other common examples of semisynthetic opioids include oxymorphone (Vicodin); oxycodone (Percocet, Roxicodone, OxyContin), which is used for pain relief; hydromorphone (Dilaudid), which is also used for pain relief; and buprenorphine (Subutex, Buprenex), which is sometimes used for pain relief but also has a large role to play in treating opioid addiction. Oxycodone, a derivative of codeine, is about one and a half times as strong as morphine in pill form. Hydromorphone, a derivative of morphine, is about four to five times as strong. Buprenorphine, a derivative of oripavine, is about 40 times as strong as morphine.

One semisynthetic opioid of special interest to paramedics and other emergency medical providers is the drug called naloxone (Narcan). Unlike the rest of the drugs discussed so far in this chapter, naloxone actually blocks the opioid receptors and blocks the effects of opioids, and it therefore works as an antidote medication to reverse opioid overdose. Being a semisynthetic opioid, it has a shape similar to other opioids, but its shape is such that it covers up the opioid receptors without actually activating these receptors. Thus, if a patient has overdosed on heroin and is given a dose of naloxone before it is too late, the naloxone can cover up the opioid receptors, block the heroin from binding, and reverse the effects of heroin. Naloxone can be injected by medical professionals into the vein or muscle. Increasingly, it can also be found in the form of a nasal spray so that it can be administered even by those who are not medical professionals.

Synthetic Opioids

Unlike the semisynthetic opioids, which were developed by slightly altering the shapes of naturally occurring, precursor molecules, the numerous synthetic opioids are drugs that were synthesized in laboratories from non-opiate molecules that nonetheless were found to be able to activate opioid receptors. Two of the most well-known synthetic opioids are called methadone and fentanyl.

Methadone is a somewhat politically controversial drug that is used in opioid replacement therapy. Methadone has a slow onset of action, which makes it less prone to cause euphoria and therefore is less addicting. It has a long duration of its effects so that it is less prone to lead to abrupt withdrawal. It also has less side effects at high doses, something that has made it useful in the treatment of both high levels of pain and in the treatment of opioid addiction. Methadone maintenance is a common strategy to transition patients away from addictions to other types of opioids.

The highly potent synthetic opioid fentanyl, as mentioned above, was developed in 1959 by Paul Janssen of Janssen Pharmaceutical for use in anesthesia and for pain control in terminally ill cancer patients who had developed tolerance for less potent opioids. Fentanyl does not come in pill form, but it exists in intravenous form and also multiple other novel forms. It is absorbable through the skin, so it is commonly made as an adhesive "transdermal patch" that one sticks to the body. It is even available as a berry-flavored lollipop lozenge on a stick (Actiq) so that the medication is absorbed through the lining of the mouth. Intravenous fentanyl, a synthetic opioid, is about 50 to 100 times as strong as intravenous morphine, and was developed medically to use with severely ill cancer patients who had developed tolerance to the less potent opioids. Unfortunately, illicit synthetic fentanyl not used for medical reasons has been increasingly produced in clandestine labs in China and Mexico in recent years. Dealers may receive this fentanyl in powder form. It can then be mixed with a diluting inert powder to decrease its potency and then sold as though it were heroin, even though the effect is not exactly the same. Powdered synthetic fentanyl can be deadly to police examining crime scenes where a dealer's operation was located, because the fentanyl powder is so potent that if a police officer even touches it with bare skin, enough can potentially absorb through the skin to cause death.

THE NATURE OF PAIN

In order to better understand the complexities surrounding the use and misuse of opioids, it is useful to consider the complexities of treating pain. Everyone has experienced pain, but what exactly is pain? It is not a tangible, visible, objective thing. Rather, pain is a subjective experience, a sensation felt by an individual person. There is no definitive test to prove whether or not a person is experiencing pain. Nevertheless, few people would be willing to say that pain is not real. In the previous section, numerous drugs were listed describing their ability to relieve pain. Various drugs were described as relieving pain twice, three times, or even 100 times as well as morphine. Does this really mean, however, that someone whose pain is relieved by morphine has 100 times less pain than someone who needs fentanyl?

It turns out that pain is a complex phenomenon that partially has to do with a person's perception of that pain. The International Association for the Study of Pain defines pain as "an unpleasant sensory and emotional experience associated with actual or potential tissue damage, or described in terms of such damage." The first part of the definition describes that pain is a sensory experience, so in that way, it is similar to the sense of feeling or hearing. The second part of the definition notes it is an emotional experience. This is clear from seeing small children's reaction to pain: a small child who accidentally falls and scrapes his or her knee on the sidewalk will almost invariably start to cry. Pain may be associated with actual damage to the body, but patients may frequently complain of pain when there is no sign of physical damage to the body. For example, back pain is one of the most common reasons to visit a doctor, but an identifiable cause is not always found. Likewise, patients may describe pains to a physician that appear to be more likely a manifestation of the patient's psychological suffering. Since all sensation is ultimately a product of our brain's interpretation of our environment, it is thought that some component of pain is therefore influenced by psychological factors. Likewise, the reverse may be true that psychological suffering may be expressed by the brain in the form of a pain or other illness in the body.

The word "pain" actually describes numerous different types of sensation. The sharp pain one feels during an injury such as breaking an arm (*mechanical pain*) is clearly different from the sting of a bee (*chemical pain*) or the burn of a sunburn (*thermal pain*). Pain in nerve tissue (*neuropathic pain*) such as by injury to the spinal cord or peripheral nerves can result in a pain that has an electrical quality to it that feels like an electrical jolt down a leg or arm. Pain felt in the internal organs (*visceral pain*) may have a dull quality or a squeezing quality. Pain may also be caused by or made worse by emotional or psychological factors that are interpreted by the brain as pain in the body (*psychosomatic pain*). In summary, different parts of the body, different types of injury, and different types of disease can all result in different types of pain. As such, different treatments are needed to treat different types of pain. Most opioids, for example, are generally not as effective for neuropathic pain as they are for mechanical pain.

Pain can also occur along different timelines and is usually classified as either acute pain or chronic pain. Definitions vary, but in general, acute pain is that which has a relatively quick onset and usually resolves in less than a month. Acute pain often has an easily identifiable source, such as a broken limb or a recent surgery. Pain that has been present for more than a month but not quite three to six months is called "subacute." Chronic pain lasts longer than three to six months. One example of chronic pain is cancer pain. Cancer can spread anywhere across the body, and when it does, it often causes pain. For example, cancer can spread to bones, causing mechanical pain, and it can also spread to tissues that impinge the nervous system, causing neuropathic pain. Other causes of chronic pain include joint pain (arthritis), muscle strain, or chronic headaches. Obese patients or patients whose muscles have grown weak can experience chronic pain when the muscles are no longer strong enough to support the skeletal frame of the body, and this can result in chronically strained muscles, bones chronically rubbing together at the joints, and nerve compression when unsupported tissues push into the nerves.

OPIOID TREATMENT FOR CHRONIC PAIN

Chronic pain can be challenging to treat. There is often not a definitive, identifiable cause, and the pain a patient experiences may be a combination of different types of pain, such as neuropathic, mechanical, visceral, or psychosomatic. Opioids may help for a time, but eventually the body gains tolerance, and so increased opioids will be needed to achieve the same pain relief. Therefore, the strength of opioid a patient requires is not only a function of how much pain she is in, but also of how much tolerance her body has built up toward opioids. For example, if an elderly patient is given opioids to treat arthritis, he will eventually need more opioids to treat the pain as tolerance develops. Meanwhile, the underlying problem of eroded or inflamed joints that are the underlying cause of the pain may still exist or even get worse. As a patient needs more and more opioids, his dependence increases, as does his risk of overdose. Furthermore, after patients have used opioids for a long time, their pain receptors may become overly sensitive, so that opioids lose some of their pain-relieving effectiveness. Additionally, if such patients stop opioids, they can actually be in greater pain than when they began opioid treatment, a state called hyperalgesia. For these reasons and more, opioids are often no longer recommended for many types of chronic pain. Alternate approaches to reduce pain are preferred, such as physical therapy, non-opioid pain relievers like nerve blocks, yoga, and psychological therapies that help patients accept the state of pain they are in.

Of note, there is a sphere of medicine in which opioid medications are irreplaceable in the treatment of chronic pain. This is called palliative care, the branch of medicine that generally deals with the patients described earlier who have incurable illnesses that have brought them near the end of their lives. Since such patients have no hope of cure, palliative care physicians work to make them feel as comfortable as possible during the time they have left. Such patients may stay in institutions called hospice centers, which are comfort centers where they can receive round-the-clock care to treat the symptoms of their worsening diseases as the end of their life approaches. Opioids are often the only types of medications that can take away their pain. They will need steadily increasing doses of these medications, but since they are at the end of their lives, they are not at risk for addiction. These are exactly the patients for whom such drugs as fentanyl were designed.

Proper treatment of pain with opioids is a highly controversial topic and is crucial for understanding the opioid epidemic. This subject will be explored more in Chapters 6–8.

DANGERS OF OPIOIDS

In reference to the use of opioid medications in the treatment of chronic pain in non-terminally ill patients, CDC director Dr. Tom Frieden wrote in the *New England Journal of Medicine* in 2016, "We know of no other medication routinely used for a nonfatal condition that kills patients so frequently." Physicians have a duty to treat pain, and yet at the same time, physicians and patients need to understand that there is a duty to balance the need to treat pain with the duty to "do no harm" to patients, as per the Hippocratic oath. The greatest dangers associated with use of opioid medications are risk of overdose, risk of addiction, and risks associated with intravenous drug use for those who inject the drugs.

OPIOID OVERDOSE

Prescription opioids are the number one cause of drug overdose deaths in the United States. Opioid overdose produces a readily recognizable constellation of symptoms including confusion, vomiting, pinpoint pupils, sleepiness, loss of consciousness, slowed or stopped breathing, cold and clammy skin, and blue skin around the lips and fingernails. A major reason people die during opioid overdose is because, much like benzodiazepines, opioids decrease the brain's respiratory drive. Even after most of the blood's oxygen content has been used up, the brain that has overdosed on opioids does not sense the low oxygen content, and the person does not feel the need to breathe. Since opioid overdose results in sleepiness or loss of consciousness, the user will have no awareness he or she is not breathing, and blood oxygen levels will rapidly drop. In the absence of oxygen, the brain begins to die after only six minutes.

Why are opioid drugs so much more likely to result in overdose than other drugs? One reason is that such a wide variety of potencies and formulations exist. This makes it easy to take a more powerful opioid than one intended. One example of this involves the heavily misused prescription drug OxyContin. OxyContin, introduced in 1995 by Purdue Pharmaceuticals, is an extended-release form of the semisynthetic opioid drug oxycodone. Most prescription opioid drugs have a relatively short duration of action in the body, and so patients may need to take another dose every four to six hours to control pain. OxyContin, however, is an oxycodone pill produced in such a way that the drug is released slowly into the body to last for 12 hours. Unfortunately, OxyContin became notorious in the early 2000s for its misuse when it became known among users that crushed or broken pills would release all the oxycodone rapidly. Thus, rapid release of a drug that was supposed to release slowly over 12 hours allowed for greater potency, greater highs, and also greater overdose risk.

A more recent example of the way that the wide variety of potencies of opioids can lead to overdose involves the synthetic opioid fentanyl. Due to its high potency and its relatively low cost to make, fentanyl has become a favorite among drug dealers. Heroin dealers who wish to stretch out their inventory will cut their heroin by mixing in a small amount of fentanyl and also other powdery substances such as flour or chalk; this way they can make it appear they are selling more heroin than they are. However, since fentanyl is so potent, it is easy for a dealer to overestimate how much fentanyl to mix with the cut heroin, and the result is that the user overdoses. As a result, fentanyl has been responsible for an increasingly large number of overdose deaths. Nearly half of all heroin deaths between 2012 and 2014 were associated with fentanyl. Heroin users are not the only ones at risk of fentanyl overdose. There have been cases of lab analyses that have shown that street versions of counterfeit Xanax, oxycodone, and OxyContin were actually made of fentanyl.

Tolerance is another reason it is so easy to overdose on opioids. It is not uncommon for users who have built a high tolerance to opioids to overdose after detoxing from opioids. When users who have detoxed later relapse into opioid misuse, they often return to using the large doses of opioids they used before getting detoxed. If their tolerance has decreased following the detox, they won't be able to tolerate the large doses they used to, and they can overdose.

RISKS OF INTRAVENOUS DRUG USE

Another aspect of opioid misuse that makes it so dangerous is the tendency for users to gravitate toward injecting the drugs directly into the vein. Users often prefer intravenous (directly into a vein) injection of opioids because this allows for the quickest uptake into the body and also ensures the greatest possible amount of the drug reaches the bloodstream (and therefore the brain). This was seen in the example of intravenous morphine being three times as potent as morphine swallowed in pill form. Use of intravenous drugs, however, is associated with numerous increased risks, such as scar formation, collapsing of veins, and contracting deadly viral or bacterial infections. Needle sharing is responsible for the spread of many infections between users. One of the most common ways that HIV is transmitted in the United States is by the spread of the virus among intravenous drug users who are sharing needles. Hepatitis C, a virus that can cause liver failure and death, is also commonly spread through needle sharing. Other types of infection are increased for intravenous drug users. Even if the needle is sterile, each skin puncture is an opportunity for bacteria from the skin to infect the wound. Bacteria living on the skin can seed into the bloodstream when the skin is broken by the needle. The more times a user breaks the skin with the needle, the higher the odds of getting such an infection. Abscesses filled with pus can form around the injection site and can even turn to gangrene. Bacterial infections of the blood can cause a condition called septic shock in which the blood pressure drops rapidly. Without blood pressure, the blood cannot pump through the veins, and death can occur. Bacteria entering the bloodstream in this way also increases risk for contracting a deadly infection of the heart called endocarditis that can eat away at the heart's internal structures.

Opioid Dependence and Withdrawal

People who become addicted to opioids and want to escape often have an extraordinarily difficult time doing so. Two of the major reasons for this are the development of psychological dependence and physiological dependence.

Psychological dependence can make it extraordinarily easy to relapse after an attempt to quit. Chronic use of opioids creates changes in the structure of the brain. As a result, people who become addicted to opioids will usually face a lifetime of cravings and compulsions to use, especially when they encounter people or places associated with their prior use. This is likely due to opioids' direct stimulation of the dopamine reward pathways, which results in long-term cravings and thought patterns that are not seen in benzodiazepines. (This is also one of the reasons that barbiturates have been almost totally replaced by benzodiazepines, since the barbiturates more often resulted in long-term cravings.)

Physiological dependence also creates a barrier to sobriety because of the uncomfortable withdrawal symptoms that develop if patients stop taking the drugs. Withdrawal from opioids produces a very specific and recognizable syndrome of symptoms that are more or less the opposite of what one would see in an overdose of opioids. Symptoms usually begin 6 to 12 hours after the last dose of a short-acting opioid or 30 hours after the last dose of a long-acting opioid. Patients can experience nausea, vomiting, stomach pains, diarrhea, restlessness, anxiety, irritability, joint pain, bone pain, yawning, tremor, dilated pupils, drug cravings, and goosebumps, in which the patient's body hairs stand up straight. These symptoms usually peak at about 72 hours and then last about a week in total. Opioid withdrawal is very uncomfortable, but unlike withdrawal from benzodiazepines or alcohol, it is not deadly. As was shown in the previous chapter, detoxifying from benzodiazepines can be deadly due to possible asphyxiation during seizure activity. The same is true for alcohol withdrawal. Fortunately, no such seizure risk exists in opioid withdrawal. Nevertheless, the symptom burden is heavy enough to be a significant barrier to cessation of opioid use.

Opioid Detox and Replacement Therapies

In order to ease the withdrawal symptoms of opioids, patients can seek to detox or wean themselves from the drug by using tapered doses of methadone or buprenorphine/naloxone that decrease by a small amount each day. Detox is essentially a treatment for physical dependence.

Methadone is a synthetic opioid that has unique properties that are useful in opioid detoxification. Due to its long duration of action in the body, methadone hangs around longer in the body, and compared to shorter-acting opioids, it exits the body more gradually. Methadone doesn't have the uneven peaks and valleys of blood concentration that are found when taking short-acting opioids like oxycodone pills or morphine pills. This long duration of action keeps the body from experiencing abrupt drops in opioid concentrations, giving it time to slowly readjust while keeping withdrawal symptoms in check. Methadone is also a good choice for detoxification compared with many other opioids because patients are less likely to get high from methadone. Studies have shown that the high, or euphoria feeling, that people get from opioids is largely an effect of the rate in which the opioid floods the system. One reason that heroin is thought to be so popular and pleasurable is because when injected, it fills the opioid receptors in the reward center of the brain more quickly than other opioids. Methadone, on the other hand, when taken orally, slowly gets absorbed into the bloodstream. In this way, it does not produce the high of heroin or other opioids, and yet it fills the opioid receptors long enough that the person does not experience withdrawal symptoms.

Methadone maintenance therapy is a system by which those who have developed an opioid addiction can receive daily doses of methadone from a methadone clinic. The giving of methadone at these clinics is highly monitored. Early on in treatment, the patients may need to come to the methadone clinic every day in order to get their daily dose. They must be observed swallowing the methadone. They cannot take it home until trust has been built, since methadone has a certain street value. (Methadone has more euphoric effects when it is injected instead of taken orally.) Patients are generally required to follow up with addiction specialists at regular intervals and are usually required to do regular drug tests. As patients continue to follow the rules, they can gain increasing levels of trust and be able to get multiple doses of methadone at a time so that they can take it home and not have to come to the clinic so often.

Methadone maintenance is sometimes controversial and is often stigmatized in the general public, since the view is held that methadone maintenance is simply "replacing one addiction for another" when abstinence should be the goal. Residents of a neighborhood also may not want to live near a methadone clinic due to the perception that they serve as magnets for "junkies" and criminals. However, for many who suffer from opioid addiction, methadone maintenance may be the best hope. Methadone maintenance in a properly monitored facility is certainly safer than illicit drug use. No other method has been shown to result in lower relapse rates.

Another, increasingly popular drug for use in detoxification and for replacement therapy is the combination drug Suboxone. Suboxone is actually two drugs in one: buprenorphine and naloxone. It is usually manufactured in the form of a small rectangular film that is placed under the tongue and absorbed from there into the blood. Buprenorphine is a unique opioid that is a useful replacement to help wean patients off opioids. It works so well for this purpose because it has a "ceiling" to its effectiveness. After doses of buprenorphine are increased to a certain level, the euphoric and respiratory depressing effects of buprenorphine do not continue to increase. Thus, even if the dose is further increased past this level, the effect of the drug remains no higher than it was at the ceiling dose. Therefore, it is less susceptible to abuse, since its effects can only go so high. The addition of naloxone is another reason Suboxone is so useful for opioid replacement therapy. As noted earlier in this chapter, naloxone is an antidote to opioid overdose, and it works by blocking the opioid receptors. Naloxone as part of Suboxone is used to prevent users from crushing it up and injecting it into their veins all at one time in pursuit of a more potent burst of buprenorphine. When a patient places the Suboxone film under his or her tongue, the body absorbs a smooth stream of buprenorphine into the blood. The naloxone is left behind and does not get absorbed under the tongue, due to its different molecular properties from buprenorphine. If the Suboxone is injected into the vein, the naloxone will enter the bloodstream at the same time as the buprenorphine, and the naloxone will then block all the opioid receptors, preventing the buprenorphine having an effect and possibly causing opioid withdrawal. This prevents misuse of the drug.

CHAPTER 5

"Uppers" and Performance Enhancers: Stimulants and Related Drugs

Stimulants, or "uppers," are valued medically and nonmedically for their ability to increase wakefulness, focus, concentration, and motivation. As opposed to the "downer" drugs that slow the activity level of the brain, such as benzodiazepines or opioids, stimulant drugs are used to increase the level of arousal in the nervous system. Stimulants also provide a euphoric effect, stimulating the same reward pathway as other addictive drugs. As a result, stimulants can be used recreationally to provide euphoria as well as increased mental energy and wakefulness. Prescription stimulants such as amphetamine (Adderall, Dexedrine) are also frequently used nonmedically as performance enhancers, such as in school settings or athletic settings. For students wanting to achieve high grades, prescription stimulants such as Adderall (amphetamine) or Ritalin (methylphenidate) can give a large boost in motivation to study and ability to focus. For this reason, these medications are commonly referred to as "study drugs." For athletes wanting to improve their performance, stimulants can similarly provide a boost in energy and fight against fatigue. Misuse of amphetamines frequently occurs in the working world among truck drivers who need help staying awake on long journeys. Likewise, amphetamines are popular among people working in business or other industries with deadlines to be met.

Stimulants are used medically for multiple different diseases and disorders, including attention deficit hyperactivity disorder (ADHD), narcolepsy, chronic fatigue syndrome, refractory depression, obesity, impulse control disorders, asthma, nasal congestions, anesthesia, and more. Some of the most well-known stimulants used in medicine are amphetamine (prescribed as Adderall and often used in the treatment of ADHD), methylphenidate (Ritalin; another common treatment for ADHD), cocaine (sometimes used as a local anesthetic), and pseudoephedrine (Sudafed; over-the-counter medication used to treat nasal congestion). Even meth-amphetamine, most often thought of as an illicit drug produced in sketchy illegal laboratories, is still technically available as a prescribed substance for use in ADHD, although the stigma of the drug is now so high that it has become rare for doctors to actually do so.

A list of some prescription and over-the-counter stimulant drugs is here:

Amphetamines and amphetamine-like substances:

- Dextroamphetamine (Dexedrine)
- Amphetamine salts (Adderall)
- Lisdexamphetamine (Vyvanse)
- Methylphenidate (Ritalin, Concerta)
- Dexmethylphenidate (Focalin)
- Methamphetamine (Desoxyn)
- Ephedrine: previously available as a diet supplement for weight loss, FDA stopped its sale for this purpose in 2006; still available over the counter for congestion and other purposes, but its availability varies by state
- Pseudoephedrine (Sudafed): sold over the counter but customers are limited in how much they can buy because it can be used to make methamphetamine
- Modafinil (Provigil)
- Propylhexedrine (Benzedrex)
- Bupropion (Wellbutrin): Prescribed more for antidepressant effects than stimulant effects
- Phenylpropanolamine (PPA): Not able to be prescribed since 2005 due to unacceptably dangerous side effects

Cocaine and cocaine analogs:

- Cocaine is no longer used in medicine as a stimulant, only as a local anesthetic.
- Other cocaine analogs are also not generally used for stimulant effects but may be used in other areas of medicine.

In terms of illegal use, the most widely used psychoactive drugs after cannabis are the amphetamines. "Amphetamines" as a group is the broad name for a larger class of drugs that derive from or are similar to the molecule amphetamine. For example, methamphetamine, the drug featured heavily in the hit TV show *Breaking Bad*, is essentially an amphetamine molecule that has had an extra branch of atoms added to it ($-CH_3$). Street names for various amphetamines include "speed," "ice," "chalk," "crystal," "crystal meth," and "meth." Numerous illegal, recreational designer drugs listed as Schedule I controlled substances and not considered to have medical use are also chemically similar to amphetamine. For example, MDMA (3,4-Methylenedioxymethamphetamine, also known by its slang terms "ecstasy," "E," or "molly"), is structurally quite similar to amphetamine.

Although cocaine is used in medical settings, its legal, prescription form is not generally considered a major contributor to the greater problem of cocaine abuse in the United States, for which the supply is almost exclusively sourced from the black market.

EFFECTS OF STIMULANTS ON THE BRAIN AND NERVOUS SYSTEM

To understand the phenomenology—that is, the first-person experience—of taking a CNS stimulant, it is instructive to consider the effects of caffeine. Caffeine is a common mild stimulant and one of the most widely used psychoactive substances in the world. When a person ingests caffeine, there can be pleasurable effects including a feeling of increased wakefulness, increased focus, and increased well-being. Caffeine is a naturally occurring compound found in coffee seeds, tea leaves, and kola nuts. These caffeine-producing plants have in turn been made into some of the most popular beverages on the planet: coffee, tea, and Coca-Cola. Both coffee and tea have been drunk for centuries for their stimulant properties. Coffee is made from the roasted seeds of the *coffea* genus of plants, which are native to parts of Africa and Asia; and in 2017, 64% of all adults in the United States drank at least one cup of coffee every day. Over half of all adults in the United States drink tea each day, often in the form of iced tea. Other psychostimulant drugs, both prescription and nonprescription, produce an effect that is more or less in the same vein as the effect produced by coffee, but the more potent stimulants give a much more profound feeling of wakefulness and focus, and they can be much more euphoric. As with other substances, the feeling of euphoria is generally the marker of possible addiction, since users can seek to recapture this rewarding feeling. Likewise, many stimulant drugs carry much greater risks and more dangerous side effects than what are found in coffee.

Unlike the downer drugs, which act as CNS depressants, the stimulant drugs actually increase the activity of the sympathetic nervous system, and therefore increase the brain and body's arousal. They are often called "sympathomimetics" in that they somewhat mimic the effects of the sympathetic nervous system. In general, stimulants increase the levels of norepinephrine and dopamine in the brain. They generally accomplish this by mechanisms that cause norepinephrine and dopamine molecules to remain longer in the synapses between neurons. Norepinephrine (also known as noradrenaline) is one of the molecules produced by the body to signal fight-or-flight mode, as was discussed in Chapter 3. Dopamine increases motivation and feelings of well-being. When these chemicals are left floating around in the synapse, it gives them increased time to interact with the nerve cells and therefore cause a more potent effect. Individual stimulants vary in the amount of each that they help release into the brain, and they vary in where they are released in the brain. In a sense, these drugs can bring users more into the fight-or-flight mode so that they reach the level of arousal needed to complete tasks set before them. More blood rushes to the brain and the skeletal muscles, so that more energy can be spent on focusing the brain. If you are an athlete, this redirection of blood to your brain and to your skeletal muscles means you can exercise longer and still feel less fatigued. (Use of many stimulants are therefore banned from professional sporting competitions unless the athlete has a legal prescription.)

Dopamine and norepinephrine released by stimulants have different effects in the brain than when dopamine is released after taking a medication like oxycodone. This is because stimulant medications cause dopamine and norepinephrine (noradrenaline) to be released into different parts of the brain than opioids do. The brain is organized anatomically, and different physical locations of the brain are associated with different mental functions. For example, the left side of the brain is in general more used for analytical and mathematical functions, while the right side of the brain is more responsible for language and visual-spatial functions. The cerebellum is the part of the brain that controls balance and coordination. The specific anatomical area of the brain where stimulants may produce the greatest effect to increase focus is called the prefrontal cortex. The prefrontal cortex is the area of the brain closest to the forehead, and this is where many of the brain's "executive functions" are performed, meaning this is the area of the brain where mental functions such as organizing, planning, and attention are primarily located. In Chapter 2, the function of dopamine was discussed in terms of its role as a neurotransmitter in the part of the brain called the mesolimbic dopamine circuit, also known as the "final common pathway of reward." When a drug such as oxycodone causes dopamine to be released into that part of the brain, it has been shown that this burst of dopamine directly causes the feeling of euphoria experienced with all addictive substances of abuse. Likewise, a stimulant such as amphetamine also causes a release of dopamine release into this reward circuit, which accounts for its abuse potential, but in addition, amphetamine also causes a release of dopamine (and norepinephrine) into a structure called the mesocortical pathway, a neural circuit that flows from the midbrain into the prefrontal cortex. In this pathway, dopamine is used as a neurotransmitter whose job is to mediate the high-level executive functions of the prefrontal cortex, like planning, motivation, and attention. This explains why many stimulant medications are often so effective for ADHD, since increased dopamine in this pathway increases the brain's ability to perform these high-level functions.

A Brief History of Amphetamines and Other Stimulants

The use of plants containing stimulant molecules dates back thousands of years. In China, the plant species *ephedra sinica*, also known by its Chinese name ma-huang, has been used in Chinese medicine for over 5,000 years for its stimulant and therapeutic effects. In 1887, a Japanese chemist named Nagai Nagayoshi first isolated the chemical responsible for ma-huang's effects. This chemical is called ephedrine, and it is still used to this day in numerous countries, particularly to prevent low blood pressure during spinal anesthesia. (Additionally, ephedrine was previously available in the United States as a weight loss drug, though this was discontinued in the United States in 2006 due to dangerous side effects and abuse potential.) Coincidentally, 1887 was the same year that German scientist Lazar Edethe first synthesized the amphetamine molecule. The amphetamine molecule was not known at that time to have medicinal or stimulant use, and there was little interest in it until around 1927, when American scientist Gordon Alles resynthesized the molecule and was the first to describe its mental effects. In 1933, the pharmaceutical company Smith, Kline, and French began selling an inhaled version of amphetamine called Benzedrine for use as a decongestant and for asthma. A pill form of Benzedrine was introduced three years later and was used to treat a variety of illnesses such as narcolepsy, postencephalitic parkinsonism, depression, and lethargy. Amphetamine quickly became popular in the medical community as well as with the general public. Amphetamine pills were used widely in World War II to help soldiers fight off hunger and fatigue. They were colloquially called "go pills." Sadly, the German army provided amphetamine pills to soldiers in the Panzer division to help them stay awake during the initial surprise Blitzkrieg attacks on western European countries such as France. Later in the 1940s and 1950s, university students slowly realized that Benzedrine inhalers could be taken apart to reveal a paper strip containing amphetamine, and chewing on this or swallowing it gave a euphoric and stimulant effect. These inhalers became popular recreational drugs, allowing users to stay awake into late hours, and they were fondly called "bennies." Benzedrine inhalers were banned in 1959, and amphetamine was limited to prescription use. Amphetamine is best known today as the prescription drug Adderall, used as treatment for ADHD. Following the discontinuation of the Benzedrine inhaler, university students have continued their use of amphetamine in the form of Adderall as both a party drug and a study drug. The stimulant methylphenidate (Ritalin) is also widely used in this way. Students today commonly receive Adderall, Ritalin, or other ADHD medications from their peers who have ADHD. Students with ADHD on prescription stimulants may offer extra pills for sale over social media or to their friends by word of mouth. They are often diverted in small quantities in this way between friends rather than through a more established drug dealer. Students may take the pills orally, or sometimes the instant-release formulations (as opposed to the extended-release formulations) are crushed up and snorted nasally. In addition to the common diversion of these medications for cognitive performance enhancement, amphetamine and methylphenidate are also frequently used as club drugs and for rave parties, where they allow users to stay awake dancing for long hours.

Methamphetamine has a somewhat parallel history to that of amphetamine. Methamphetamine was first synthesized in Japan in 1893 by Nagai Nagayoshi, the same chemist who first isolated ephedrine from ma-huang. The methamphetamine molecule was found to have even more potent and longer-lasting effects as amphetamine, and it was produced heavily in Japan in the 1920s for use as a stimulant, for a diet aid, and for opening airways in the lungs. Much like amphetamine has been used in wartime, methamphetamine was used by Japanese pilots in WWII before embarking on kamikaze flights to give them the aggression and self-confidence to undertake their missions. In the United States, the FDA approved methamphetamine in 1944 for treatment of narcolepsy, mild depression, postencephalitic Parkinsonism, chronic alcoholism, hay fever, and obesity. It was originally sold legally as an over-the-counter drug called methedrine and was marketed to housewives to help fight depression and weight gain, truck drivers to help stay awake, students to increase intellectual function, and athletes wanting to increase physical performance. In the United States, methamphetamine pills are currently still approved by the FDA for only two indications, ADHD and obesity. In practice, however, it is not widely prescribed by physicians due to the great stigma attached. Illegal production of methamphetamine for recreational use in the United States often occurs in small, secret laboratories using various production methods. One method involves the use of the molecule called pseudoephedrine, which is the active ingredient in the nonprescription nasal decongestant drug Sudafed. Producers can easily convert pseudoephedrine into methamphetamine in their labs to sell in the black market. Medications containing pseudoephedrine used to be sold over the counter in the United States until Congress passed the Combat Methamphetamine Epidemic Act of 2005. Although it is still legal to purchase medications with pseudoephedrine without a prescription, it has now moved "behind-the-counter" so that purchasers must now show identification in order to buy. The government tracks how many boxes of this medication a person buys, and each person is only allowed a set rationed number of boxes per month.

The medical history of amphetamines is still being written. Although MDMA is still currently a Schedule I drug, and thus is not currently available by prescription or considered acceptable for medical use, this classification may change over the next several years. The FDA has given approval to researchers to perform a large-scale, Phase III clinical trial of MDMA to test its safety and efficacy for use as a treatment for PTSD (post-traumatic stress disorder) in conjunction with talk therapy to help those who suffer from the disorder to be able to open up, process the trauma, and find relief. Though structurally similar to amphetamine, MDMA has increased action at the serotonin receptor, in addition to action at the dopamine and norepinephrine receptors. In addition to stimulatory effects, MDMA has slight psychedelic effects and is known to increase sociability and feelings of connectedness with others. The idea behind the current research on MDMA for the treatment of PTSD is that the feelings of empathy and connectedness that MDMA causes might serve as a way to help those suffering from PTSD to open up and feel increased safety with a therapist to facilitate discussing their traumas, allowing them to accelerate the rate of therapy and healing in order to better process and integrate the traumatic memories and thus decrease PTSD symptoms such as flashbacks, hypervigilance, and nightmares.

Another stimulant used widely since antiquity is cocaine. Cocaine is derived from coca leaves that are indigenous to South America. Coca leaves are not from one specific plant but rather can be leaves from any one of four different coca plants belonging to a family of plant species called the *erythroxylaceae*. These leaves have been chewed for millennia, particularly in Peru by native peoples such as the Inca, as far back as 3,000 BCE for their ability to fight fatigue and suppress the appetite. The coca leaf's use in the West did not become popular until the 1800s, however, because the coca leaves did not retain their potency when shipped on long voyages across the ocean. Finally, in 1860, German chemist Albert Niemann described the isolation of pure cocaine from the coca leaf. In 1862, Merck began selling cocaine to researchers. Interest in the drug started to explode around this time. Sigmund Freud, one of the most important figures in psychology and the father of psychoanalysis, was known to be an avid cocaine user for many years until he came to understand its high potential for addiction. Originally trained as a medical doctor, Freud wrote a review paper in 1884 about cocaine called "Uber Coca" in which he touted the numerous medical and mental benefits of the drug. Around the same time, a French pharmacist named Angelo Mariani patented a beverage that combined cocaine extract and Bordeaux wine, which was called Vin Mariani. This cocaine-containing alcoholic beverage became so popular internationally, it was even given a glowing endorsement by Pope Leo XIII. Mariani received a gold medal from the Vatican for inventing the beverage, and the pope's accolades even went so far that he agreed to give his endorsement in a print advertisement for the company, allowing his photo to be used for this purpose. Around the same time that Vin Mariani was being invented and sold, a pharmacist named John Pemberton of Atlanta, Georgia, began perfecting the recipe for another cocaine-containing beverage that would become immensely popular, Coca-Cola. This drink originally included the two stimulants cocaine and caffeine (derived from the kola nut). The cocaine was eventually removed in 1903, but the reference to the coca leaf has always remained in the drink's name. Cocaine thus enjoyed wide popularity during the late nineteenth and early twentieth century. It was sold widely in the United States on the black market but also for a time in the form of commercially produced, unregulated over-the-counter "patent medications." The drug was used increasingly for recreational purposes until 1920 or so, when its use began to decline as the public became more wary of its ill effects. Its popularity only resurged in the 1970s and 1980s, possibly because the prior generations who had become skeptical of the drug had largely died off by that time. In the late 1980s, cocaine in the form of "crack" became more popular because of its increased potency, higher even than the powdered form of the drug. (Inhaled drugs have the fastest route to the brain and produce greater highs than other forms of administration, even more so than injecting or snorting the drug). Cocaine's accepted legitimate medical uses have dwindled greatly over the past century. It is no longer used medically for its stimulant properties, but its use continues for its properties as a local anesthetic in some surgeries of the eyes and nose because it numbs pain at the same time as it dilates blood vessels, a property useful for surgeries involving delicate structures such as the tear ducts, which need to ensure a steady blood supply.

Cathinone and its related molecules are another major group of naturally occurring stimulant molecules that are popular in certain parts of the world. The cathinone molecule closely resembles the amphetamine molecule (cathinone's other chemical name is beta-keto-amphetamine), and it is found in nature most abundantly in the leaves of a plant called *khat* or *qat* (*Catha edulis*). Khat plants are endemic to regions in the Horn of Africa, such as Ethiopia, Djibouti, and Somalia, and in the Arabian Peninsula, particularly in Yemen. The chewing of khat leaves in these countries is highly popular, due to their stimulating and euphoric effects. Khat has never been highly popular in the West as a recreational drug due to the difficulty of transporting its highly perishable leaves. Recreational use of cathinone molecules in the West most commonly occurs in the form of numerous designer drug molecules collectively known as "bath salts," which can have effects similar to other stimulants listed above. These drugs are usually produced in illegal labs and sold on the black market, and these labs are notorious for having poorly controlled processing that can leave poisonous chemical impurities in the final product. One of the most well-known molecules that was sold as bath salts is called MDPV (methylenedioxypyrovalerone). MDPV has stimulant effects similar to amphetamine or cocaine, and there are also reports it can cause drug-induced psychosis. The most famous case of bath salts psychosis occurred during the "cannibal attack" in 2012 in Miami, Florida, where a homeless man who was believed to be high on bath salts was shot and killed by police when he was found attacking and eating the face of another, living man. Before the MDPV molecule was banned by the government, it was sold legally over the counter for a time in gas stations and convenience stores.

There is a widely prescribed antidepressant and smoking cessation-aid drug called bupropion (Wellbutrin) belongs to a class of molecules called the "substituted cathinones," and it has a molecular shape that is very similar to cathinone. Fortunately, bupropion is generally safe and well tolerated by the body, and has a lower abuse potential. It does not have a reputation anything like that of bath salts. Bupropion was initially thought to have no psychostimulant effects, despite having a molecular shape similar to amphetamine and cathinone, but studies have shown that in doses higher than those normally prescribed, stimulant effects can be achieved. Another drug related to cathinone that also occurs naturally in the leaves of *khat* is called phenylpropanolamine (PPA). PPA is no longer available in the United States for medical use, but previously it was used as a nasal decongestant and weight loss drug. Unfortunately, it could cause life-threatening side effects at doses only three to four times higher than the standard dose—for example, leading to undue hypertension or stroke.

MEDICAL USES OF PRESCRIPTION STIMULANTS

Attention deficit hyperactivity disorder (ADHD) is the primary disorder for which stimulants are standard treatment. The symptoms of ADHD include chronic impulsivity, hyperactivity, and difficulty paying attention. These symptoms must have been present since childhood, with evidence of their having existed between the ages 6 and 12. These symptoms must be of such a severity as to be inconsistent with their developmental level as well as causing marked impairment in function in social, academic, and occupational settings. A somewhat controversial disorder in the eyes of the general public, who sometimes view it as simply normal childhood behavior, ADHD is well established within the medical community and is the most highly studied and diagnosed mental disorder in children. ADHD is a chronic condition classified as a neurodevelopmental psychiatric disorder, meaning the brains of children with ADHD show differences from those of people without ADHD. For example, children with ADHD have a reduced volume in certain areas of the brain, such as the left prefrontal cortex, which is responsible for working memory, planning, organization, and more. As with most illnesses, the cause of ADHD is thought to be a combination of genetic and environmental factors, and there is good evidence that genetics play a large role in the development of ADHD. Twin studies looking at health outcomes of identical twins who had been adopted into separate foster homes (hence, comparing children with identical genomes but raised in different environments) found that genetics account for about 75% of the expression of ADHD symptoms. Stimulant medications operating in the prefrontal cortex help to counteract the attentional deficits. At first, it may seem counterintuitive to give stimulant medications to a child who is already impulsive and hyperactive, and therefore appears to have excess mental energy. However, a major neural deficit these children face is a relatively low amount of the exact neurotransmitters that stimulant medications supply, norepinephrine and dopamine. These children actually lack the mental energy to sustain attention and concentration, and so they get quickly frustrated and switch to a different, less demanding task. Stimulants replenish the neurotransmitters and give them the energy to sustain focus. Thus, paradoxically, many people with ADHD say that stimulants make them feel more "normal."

Much of the confusion among the general public is likely because the symptoms for ADHD, when read in the DSM or on a website, for example, could sound like normal childhood behavior. However, what is often difficult for the layperson to observe is that children with ADHD have attentional problems to such a greater degree than the average child that it becomes qualitatively different. An analogy for this is the way that general public often view major depressive disorder with skepticism. To the average person who has neither experienced MDD nor interacted with someone with MDD, it is easy to brush off their symptoms as phony or a lack of willpower, since everyone gets "depressed" or feels sad to a certain extent. However, most people do not ever get depressed to such a high degree that they are unable to sleep, lose 20 pounds (or more) from low appetite, lose their job because don't have the energy to get out of bed, and have a desire to take their own life. Thus the difference between normal "depressed" feelings of sadness and the depression seen in major depressive disorder is a matter of the intensity and duration of the depression. Likewise, for those who have never experienced up-close the high degree of organizational and attentive struggles that people with ADHD undergo every day, it can be difficult to understand.

What happens when the child with ADHD becomes an adult? The human brain continues to develop well into the second and third decades of life. As a result, some children diagnosed with ADHD will "grow out of" their disorder as the brain continues to develop and/or different strategies are learned to help them eventually compensate for their disorder. Nonetheless, 30 to 50% of these children will grow up and continue to have clinically significant symptoms into adulthood, causing them functional problems in school, work, relationships, and other settings. As the child ages, the disorder often eventually becomes an "invalidating disorder" in that the person can be told negative things about themselves for years such as that he or she is lazy or stupid (as opposed to suffering from an attention deficit). This can lead to profound damage to a person's self-esteem, which in turn can lead to comorbid conditions such as depressive disorders, anxiety disorders, addictions, and personality disorders.

Multiple prescription stimulants are used in the treatment of ADHD. The first-line choices for medical treatments of ADHD are generally Adderall or Ritalin. These also exist in extended-release versions that last all day, as neither drug lasts all day in its immediate-release form. Another popular ADHD drug is Vyvanse. This medication acts like an extended-release version of Adderall. Chemically, Vyvanse is essentially a molecule of amphetamine that has had an amino acid added to it. The amphetamine molecule is not active as a stimulant as long as the amino acid is bound to it. The body naturally breaks down this molecule and separates the amino acid from the amphetamine molecule slowly over an extended period of time. In this way, the active amphetamine molecule is slowly released into the blood. Thus, it is thought that Vyvanse has less abuse potential since it does not rush as quickly to the brain and produces less euphoria. In addition to medications, treatment of ADHD also includes counseling and lifestyle changes to help manage symptoms.

Stimulants also have medical use in the treatment of narcolepsy. Narcolepsy is a neurological disorder where a person has periods of excessive sleepiness during the day due to a disruption in the sleep-wake cycle. They may also have periods called "cataplexy" in which they experience sudden loss of muscle strength, causing for example, dropping of the jaw, buckling of the knees, and neck weakness. The decreased muscle strength may transition into sleepiness and spontaneous episodes of sleep. These episodes are often triggered by strong emotional reactions, such as when the person experiences sudden anger, embarrassment, laughter, awe, or surprise. Stimulants, particularly modafinil or adrafinil, are used in patients with narcolepsy to promote wakefulness.

STIMULANT SIDE EFFECTS AND TOXICITY

Prescription stimulants have similar side effect profiles, as most have a similar mechanism of action in the body and are related to amphetamines. Amphetamines used medically are usually tolerated well at the normal prescribed dosages. Common side effects are insomnia, anxiety, dysphoria, irritability, fast heart rate, increased blood pressure, and heart palpitations. Less commonly, patients might experience movement disorders such as motor tics or symptoms of Tourette's syndrome. These symptoms usually go away after 7 to 10 days. They may exacerbate patients' preexisting disorders, such as glaucoma, hyperthyroidism, hypertension, seizure disorders, anxiety disorders, and psychotic disorders. High doses can cause dry mouth, dilated pupils, teeth-grinding, restlessness, seizures, and mood swings. Overt psychosis can also occur at high doses, resulting in symptoms such as hallucinations and paranoia. It is thought that long-term use of amphetamines can cause a delusional disorder similar to schizophrenia. There is evidence that stimulants can slow growth in children. Overdose of amphetamines can lead to dangerously high blood pressure, dangerously fast heart rate, failure of the heart to pump blood, bleeding into the brain, compulsive and repetitive movement, agitation, muscle breakdown, elevated body temperature, urinary retention, and more. Overdose of prescription stimulants is much more rare than that of prescription opioids or benzodiazepines. Dependence on amphetamines at medically prescribed doses is rare. They are generally thought not to be as addictive as opioids or even benzodiazepines. There is a withdrawal syndrome with amphetamines, but it is much milder than what is found with opioids, benzodiazepines, and alcohol, and generally is not fatal. The most common symptoms of amphetamine withdrawal are fatigue and increased appetite. However, the abuse potential of these medications is still high, and there is significant risk of diversion and resale of prescriptions.

PART II

Issues and Controversies

CHAPTER 6

The Business of Medicine

The opioid crisis didn't appear overnight, and didn't arise in a vacuum. As with many nonnatural disasters, the road to this crisis was paved with good intentions. Regulatory agencies such as the United States Food and Drug Administration, scientific research and peer-reviewed journal publications, the judicial system, and even those having taken the Hippocratic oath, failed to protect Americans from malicious greed and showed little appetite to reform even after that failure was publicized. I highly recommend to anyone wishing for a deep understanding of this crisis and the interplay of pharmaceutical companies, physicians, and drug traffickers *Dream Land* by Sam Quinones. No book about this epidemic has combined compassion for victims with tenacious reporting like Quinones has.

Opioids were first discovered around 3400 BCE in Southwest Asia, in an innocuous, pretty flower called the opium poppy, although locals called it the "joy plant." Its painkilling properties became valued, then commercialized, spreading through Europe and beyond, eventually becoming a featured product along the ancient trade route known as the Silk Road. Long before the War on Drugs, opium started two separate wars, colloquially called the Opium Wars, in the nineteenth century. They arose as a result of British sellers smuggling and trading opium in China, resulting in close to 12 million Chinese addicted individuals. It was the first drug-trafficking operation on a large international scale, and despite pleas from the Chinese emperor, little could be done to staunch the tide. Profits were too great to be swayed by moral arguments, and profits lost from Chinese government seizure of opium trunks induced war. Ultimately, China was forced to appease the British by keeping the drug passageways open. These wars, which were seemingly unconnected to the United States when they were fought, would become an integral part of U.S. drug history. Toward the end of the nineteenth century, the development of the Western frontier of the United States would be powered by workers who immigrated from China. Addictions that were formed in mainland China did not cease to exist when the laborers arrived in the United States.

Morphine, the active ingredient of opium, was first extracted from opium in the early 1800s and touted as a miracle drug. The patented process through which morphine could be extracted provided the financial backing for what is today one of the largest pharmaceutical companies in the world, Merck. It became routinely prescribed by physicians for its astounding painkilling properties.

On the heels of the extraction of morphine, other pharmaceutical companies looked for their own entryway to this new class of medications. In 1874, diacetylmorphine was first synthesized by C. R. Alder Wright from morphine, and was discovered to be far more potent than morphine and hailed as a wonder drug in clinical trials. Using its chemical name, the synthesis of diacetylmorphine may not seem like such a terrible step in history. Many people, though, reported that taking the medications made them feel "heroic." The combined effects of being calm and feeling no pain led Bayer to name diacetylmorphine "heroin" in 1898.

While Merck was built on the fortune morphine produced, heroin quickly became the number one best seller for Bayer, even surpassing aspirin. By 1910, however, the grim true picture of heroin emerged. Physicians and patients began to realize that tolerance to heroin was quickly acquired by the human body. Tolerance meant that the patient needed to take more and more just to achieve the same effects a previously lower dose achieved.

Despite this emerging truth, Bayer continued its aggressive marketing. Hundreds of clinical papers extorted heroin's effectiveness. *The Boston Medical and Surgical Journal* even stated, "Heroin possesses many advantages. It's not hypnotic and there's no danger of acquiring a habit." Despite the published claims to the contrary, heroin's notoriety as a narcotic spread, which increased abuse by many people addicted to morphine and looking for an over-the-counter replacement. Even in 1912, Bayer promoted heroin products such as cough and bronchitis medicine for children, and heroin salts and lozenges aimed at a number of other maladies and illnesses. While officials were uneasy regarding morphine addiction amongst its war veterans and the damaging nature of opium usage amongst the populace, action to limit their use was slowed because at the time opium and heroin were extremely effective in relieving suffering in one of the deadliest illnesses of the day—tuberculosis. By 1913, however, Bayer decided to stop producing heroin upon receiving reports of the growing heroin-related hospital admissions. While the federal government via the Harrison Narcotics Act of 1914 took steps to make heroin prescription-only in 1914, it took another 10 years until it was banned altogether.

As heroin gasped its last legal breaths, a new variant of opioid emerged, known as oxycodone. It was synthesized in 1917, and was released to U.S.

markets in 1939. It was billed as a medicine for use only for the most ill of patients—the ones suffering from cancer and the aftereffects of major surgeries. Several decades later, one company, Purdue Pharma, would take a look at this seemingly run-of-the-mill opiate, reformulate it, market it aggressively, and create today's opiate crisis.

John Purdue Gray and George Frederick Bingham founded Purdue Pharma in 1952. At the time, Purdue Pharma sold mostly earwax removal and other obscure over-the-counter medicines. Unhappy to toil in relative medical backwaters with limited profits, the company shifted its focus. In the 1960s, it acquired the rights to Valium (generically called diazepam) and hired psychiatrist and drug advertiser Arthur Sackler to market it. Sackler developed a unique marketing approach to bring Valium to the direct attention of the supplier, the physician. He was the first to use drug detailers—salespeople who would visit physicians in their offices to offer "scientific evidence" showing the effectiveness of the drugs being pushed. To reinforce his sales pitch, he developed and distributed a marketing flyer posing as a weekly medical newspaper called *The Medical Tribune*. His tactics were brilliant and successful, and Valium became the first $100 million drug. Other pharmaceutical companies took note.

Decades later, Purdue Pharma had been purchased from its original owners. The buyers were none other than Arthur, Mortimer, and Raymond Sackler.

The company developed and patented a suspended-release oxycodone pill that they dubbed OxyContin, and its cousin, MS Contin, a suspended-release morphine pill. They called OxyContin a medical marvel, a long-lasting narcotic that could ease pain for longer on smaller doses. While double-blind placebo-controlled studies (the gold standard for establishing clinical effects of a medication) indicated that extended-release caplets, such as OxyContin and MS Contin, were only as effective as already existing immediate-release morphine and oxycodone, these studies weren't widely publicized. Similarly hidden but known to Purdue was the fact that pain relief dissipated long before the 12-hour time mark, triggering withdrawal symptoms, encouraging more pill taking, and increasing tolerance. There wasn't any research performed on patients' addiction to these medications. Furthermore, the company produced not just oxycodone in 10 milligram pill forms, but they also produced pills with as much as 160 milligrams!

Despite these privately known clinical setbacks, Purdue Pharma began to aggressively market OxyContin in 1996. Their marketing approach followed in the same vein as Arthur Sackler's previous campaigns. Far from learning from the Bayer fiasco, Purdue marketed the drug directly to physicians, attempting to overcome medical bias by funding research— research that suspiciously stated that OxyContin wasn't as addictive or dangerous as previous data on morphine derivatives implied. Purdue

Pharma claimed that OxyContin was far less addictive than other narcotics. They cited a misunderstood short letter sent to the editors of the *New England Journal of Medicine* by Porter and Jick, stating "less than 1%" of opiate users become addicted. This study did not examine long-term use. To further negate physician bias against opiates, Purdue Pharma had the FDA approve a package insert that claimed that OxyContin had less potential for abuse than other opiates due to its extended-release formula— without any scientific data to back this claim. Suspiciously but not surprisingly, the FDA employee in charge of the approval process for OxyContin left to work for Purdue Pharma. Also important to the emerging epidemic, the Purdue sales force also urged physicians to prescribe OxyContin for a variety of types of pain, a serious break from the tradition to prescribe narcotics only for cancer-related or other terminal pain.

Although the medical community was wary of morphine-related compounds based on entrenched beliefs that narcotics were to be prescribed sparingly, Purdue Pharma happened to market OxyContin and MS Contin in a time when doctors were reexamining their own bias in a wave of pain research. One such doctor who would become the poster child of false prophecy mixed with greed was Russell Portenoy. Purdue Pharma paid Portenoy to promote the drug to other clinicians, and paid sales personnel by the thousands to go "door-to-door" and speak to physicians in their clinics and their private offices. They further lured doctors with paid luxury vacations that were billed as "seminars" that promoted Purdue's products. Physicians who generated high sales were in turn paid to speak to other physicians to promote the drug as well, echoing sales pitches they memorized with specious medical data to back its claims.

It worked. Sales exploded from $48 million in 1996 to $1.1 billion just four years later. Over this period, Purdue presided over 40 all-expense-paid seminars in resorts in California, Florida, and Arizona, with over 5,000 physicians and nurses in attendance. They gave out pens, notepads, office items, and even music CDs with OxyContin's brand name plastered all over them. Meanwhile, Purdue Pharma tracked physicians' data to determine all the physicians in all pain-related fields in each zip code, how these physicians prescribed, and the highest and lowest prescribers of their drug. This data was released to its sales force, who in turn received bonuses based on whether they were able to increase a particular physician's prescription rate. In 2001, Purdue Pharma distributed $40 million in bonuses to their sales force. They distributed coupons to give patients a free one week to one month's supply; 34,000 of these coupons were redeemed. Purdue's sales force doubled, as did their physician base. By marketing the drug to non-cancer-related pain, Purdue Pharma ensured a tenfold increase in OxyContin sales by 2002.

Purdue Pharma knew shortly after OxyContin's release that the drug was being abused, as was discovered later by the Justice Department.

There were official reports of pills being stolen, of pills being crushed and snorted, of pills making their way through drug pushers, of increased OxyContin-related hospital admissions, and of doctors getting paid directly by the patient to dole out prescriptions. And yet the company ignored these claims, reassuring its sales force and its physician base and reiterating erroneous data that extended-release oxycodone wasn't habit-forming. Despite nearly 117 internal memos from sales representatives documenting potential for abuse, and evidence that the Sackler family knew about these reports, Purdue didn't attempt to change their formula for years. The Sackler family became one of Forbes's wealthiest families, with a collective net worth of $13 billion.

While addiction to opioids originated far, far before OxyContin, the Opioid Policy Research Collaborative at Brandeis University concluded that it was Arthur Sackler's unique marketing onslaught that changed the way doctors prescribed medications. It was this culture of advertising, which stealthily deployed kickbacks, misinformed physicians, used targeted demographics, and advocated off-label use for its product, that generated what would become a wave of addiction that would cripple millions of people.

By 2003, the Drug Enforcement Administration took note of rising reports of abuse and Purdue Pharma's role in that abuse with their marketing strategies. Purdue Pharma itself contributed to the education of its potential for abuse to the public by posting warning labels exhorting users, "Taking broken, chewed or crushed OxyContin tablets could lead to the rapid release and absorption of a potentially toxic dose." As overdose fatalities piled up, legal pressure urged Purdue Pharma to change its formulation of the drug to reduce misuse.

Despite its popularity, pharmacies began to refuse to stock OxyContin, due to frequent robberies. A study in *The Journal of the Canadian Medical Association* found that MS Contin was the highest-priced drug sold on the street, commanding 40 times the pharmacy's price.

By 2006, Purdue's unchallenged financial success started to be impinged upon by various forces. In 2004, a lawsuit from the State of Connecticut claimed that Purdue Pharma was causing an untold number of prescriptions to be paid from the state through Medicare and Medicaid, more than its dosing parameters allowed. Lawsuits alleging Purdue Pharma's role in medical malpractice and a growing public health epidemic piled up. In 2007, Purdue paid $600 million in one of the largest settlements in history, admitting its role in deceptive marketing of their products. Since then, thousands more lawsuits have followed, and there is good reason to believe these will continue to increase. In 2010, Purdue Pharma changed its formulation of OxyContin, so that the pill cannot be crushed into a powdered form. While they announced they were doing this to stem the tide of addiction, their commitment to this claim should be questioned. They simply took the non-crush-proof pills and sold them in other countries where regulators had not yet become aware of the harm Purdue was causing.

Prescriptions of OxyContin plummeted as the public became more aware that the medication was not nearly as benign as originally claimed. And yet, skeptics pointed out that Purdue Pharma only changed their formulation shortly before the patent on the existing version of OxyContin would expire, thus creating a new patent and a new market niche. It successfully convinced the FDA to reject all generic versions, stating that to approve dangerous generic versions of oxycodone when their new pill is harder to abuse is a public health concern.

Today, despite a growing animosity toward the company in the United States, Purdue Pharma hasn't ceded the battle to prescribe opiates—it has simply moved the borders. Purdue Pharma funds physicians to give talks in China and Brazil to extol the virtues of OxyContin through a wholly owned subsidiary branch of their company called Mundipharma.

Mundipharma gives millions to doctors like Joseph Pergolizzi Jr. to lead seminars that admonish countries for "not hav[ing] all the tools you need to properly address pain." These talks do not address the addiction potential, once again sweeping aside the perilous threat of addiction and reassuring the public that opiates aren't harmful. In a new twist, commercials in Spain use models and celebrities in television ads to reach the public directly, urging them not to live with their pain and to seek medication. Since 2007, painkiller use in Spain increased by sevenfold. Thus, Purdue Pharma, with a team of other pharmaceutical companies, cements its role as provider of opiates in a culture of a sweeping opiate epidemic. In an ironic twist, Purdue Pharma currently holds a patent on a drug that claims to wean the opiate-addicted off of opiates, proving that opiates are profitable on both sides of the fence.

While the majority of the blame rests on Purdue Pharma's shoulders, the opioid epidemic could not have been sustained without the cooperation of doctors and insurance companies. Not all physicians were naively led into prescribing OxyContin without understanding the fallout. Dr. Russell Portenoy published papers that falsified data surrounding the risk of abuse for Purdue Pharma's drugs, and got paid thousands of dollars to do so. Because of his senior position at Beth Israel Medical Center, in addition to his standing as professor at Albert Einstein College of Medicine, Portenoy was considered a prime influencer, swaying the tide of medical opinion. Other doctors followed suit, getting paid lucratively for "speaking engagements," which suspiciously coincided with their number of OxyContin prescriptions.

Another way doctors found to cash in on the opiate trend was to write prescriptions to desperate people addicted to opioids. These doctors often practiced far from the elite centers of medicine, and some had run into legal problems in the past. Essentially, regardless of whether a physician was viewed as a leader or a charlatan, there was money to be made via OxyContin. Many of these non-elite doctors opened their own clinics to meet the growing demands of addicted patients. These pain clinics devolved into what's informally known as a pill mill.

The "pill mill" became the place where drug dealing and the practice of medicine intermingled to enrich the sellers and harm the consumers. The first one opened in 1979, in Portsmouth, Ohio, a town that saw a sharp decrease in blue-collar jobs as mining and manufacturing became outsourced. Many doctors walked this path reluctantly—unemployment led to more people claiming disability as a way to pay the bills—and went to doctors claiming to be in terrible pain. Pain cannot be objectively measured or calculated. Hospitals and physicians still rely on an outdated 1–10 scale, alongside rudimentary happy and sad faces, to gauge pain levels and respond accordingly. It's hard not to feel sympathy to someone crying in an office, and with insurance reimbursements diminishing, doctors had to see more patients in a day and spend less time with each. Prescribing opiates, such as OxyContin, became the easy way to resolve a patient's problem and keep them happy. But doing so would often create a kind of backlash, spreading a physician's reputation as being an easy mark. Patients would come in demanding prescriptions, and offering cash. That cash became alluring and ultimately, difficult to ignore. Initially, many must have relied on Purdue Pharma's claim of low incidence of addiction. Over time, however, the evidence must have become difficult to disregard.

More specifically, one began to see the appearance of pill mills, or clinics masquerading as a pain-management center. Often, the doctors have a shady past, and have trouble running their own practices due to personal problems, such as malpractice lawsuits, and drug and alcohol problems. These doctors prescribe pain medication with almost no diagnosis, and frequently agree to up a dosage or increase a dosage. Medical records are barely kept. Cash is the preferred method of payment, to bypass an insurance company's auditors. The business of selling prescriptions boomed, especially in economically depressed areas. Seniors sold their prescriptions or leftover pills to drug dealers to keep them afloat in retirement, and in turn drug dealers sold their pills to street users as well as patients cut off from their previous supply of OxyContin by doctors who realized they had been hoodwinked into prescribing the drug and now wished to stop playing a part in harming their patients. Waiting rooms of these pill mills filled to bursting, mostly with street users arriving at all hours. Over time, records of prescriptions led to investigations and rescinding a doctor's medical license. However, the investigations moved slowly, and many doctors ran away to exotic locales at the first sign of an inquest with millions of dollars in cash, and a wake of overdose deaths behind them.

Around this same time, another way of bringing opiates to the street emerged. With OxyContin sales booming, before the truth about the hazards of opiates were revealed, OxyContin were doled out like candy to teenagers on the football field, in high school and college sports, and to anyone with any kind of injury. Once OxyContin sales began to fall, large masses of addicted individuals remained who couldn't obtain legally prescribed medications to meet their addiction's appetite. The addictions did not go away. In this toxic environment, a few enterprising individuals from Mexico saw their opportunity.

Xalisco is a small town in the Mexican state of Nayarit, surrounded by lush, poppy-filled mountains. In the early 2000s, the town became a prime source of drug dealers who brought heroin to the streets. These dealers changed the rules of the game in a number of ways. Their heroin was pure, in a form called "black tar heroin," a black sticky substance instead of white powder cut with other chemicals that would make the heroin less potent. They employed young, hungry men with respectable reputations, bringing small bags of this heroin in their mouths across the border. Dealers were armed only with a cell phone and a smile, delivering heroin directly to a user's house. Dealers weren't allowed to use the product or to be armed, and never had more than small amounts of drugs or cash on them at any given time. They were also on salary, so they had no reason to push more drugs or move more product, which kept things nonviolent. Combined, the new rules made obtaining heroin feel like a respectable transaction instead of a dangerous enterprise, and ensured that anyone caught wouldn't face jail time. The men were friendly, calling and checking in on their "customers" frequently to make sure they were happy. Anyone not purchasing in a while—whether because of competition or because they were trying to get sober—were met with superb customer service, a few free bags making their way to their house in record time. These deals were immensely successful, wending their way through small towns in Middle America, where they weren't competing with vengeful urban gangs, cartels, and mafia connections. Their money earned was sent back to their families in Mexico, where the dollar went further to improve living conditions, which encouraged more to join the business.

Deporting a drug dealer from Xalisco would only result in numerous replacements in a constant stream over the border, and by the time a sense of the larger picture emerged, the die was cast. Millions more became addicted, and those that wanted to quit were roped back into their addiction by tools commonly deployed by free-market capitalism.

Hospitals and insurance companies didn't make it easier to quit, either. Ever mindful of the bottom line, insurance companies frequently blocked coverage to pricey painkillers that were less addictive. Morphine and its derivatives, including oxycodone, are cheap and easy to produce. Patients would complain to physicians about untreated pain, thanks to insurance denials, yielding more prescriptions to the more hazardous opiate pain-killer. In an analysis by ProPublica and the *New York Times*, only one-third of Medicare patients had access to painkillers such as Butrans, which contains buprenorphine, a must less addictive drug. Lidocaine, another nonaddictive painkiller, required prior approval for use. Private health insurance companies followed Medicare's lead. Opioids, however, were nearly always covered and most without any prior approval. Patients who try to appeal are often denied, and often give up fighting with insurance companies, who have legal teams at their disposal. In turn, insurance companies incentivize doctors to prescribe cheaper medications, and place a heavy out-of-pocket cost for nonaddictive painkillers, thus exacerbating the problem. Furthermore, insurance companies place heavy restrictions on approval for medications designed to help addicted people off their addictive substances, such as Suboxone, further alienating patients who need help.

Pharmaceutical companies and insurance companies have regulatory bodies to manage wrongful practices such as the ones that led to the opiate epidemic. However, they are also the biggest contributors to political campaigns, lending bias to legislative oversight. Grassroots organizations that attempted to rein in over-prescription of opiates were silenced by lobbyists such as the Pain Care Forum, which spent $740 million to override attempts to cap opiate prescriptions. Purdue Pharma and other pain-medication producers spent over $900 million between 2006 and 2015 on political contributions. It's hard to track how pharmaceutical corporations and insurance companies donate money to politicians, because it's often cloaked under individual names that aren't necessarily associated with the company, or via gifts or experiences that aren't linked to a price tag.

Hospitals could not escape being part of the opiate epidemic because of a new system of rating patient care—one that measures patient satisfaction. In the early 2000s, the Center for Medicare and Medicaid Services (CMS) created the Hospital Consumer of Healthcare Providers and Systems (HCAHPS) survey that measured patient satisfaction as a way of ranking hospitals for quality of care. The Deficit Reduction Act of 2005 made the survey mandatory by imposing a penalty for not submitting their data. Another act, the Patient Protection and Affordable Care Act of 2010, made the data from the HCAHPS worth 30% of the overall hospital grade, and based reimbursement on the hospital's grade.

The flaw in this plan is that, as a measuring tool of medical success, the patient satisfaction model is a poor one. It's a subjective perspective—any toddler will argue that they hate the doctor because they received a shot, and yet vaccines are arguably vital for overall health. Patient satisfaction is often a reflection of pain and lack thereof, which they then use as a testament to how well their treatment went. In fact, there are multiple questions on the survey directly related to pain and how well it was reduced during the course of their stay. This pressured physicians to address pain foremost, sometimes at the expense of the overall health of the patient. Poor scores were often due to a denial of opiates upon request and penalized responsible physicians, obstructing their mobility in their career at the hospital. In short, these patient satisfaction surveys were unhealthily tied to hospital reimbursements, instead of directing rewards for positive medical outcomes. Multiple studies confirm this, citing that patient satisfaction scores have no correlative relationship with positive medical outcomes. Still, the patient satisfaction model continues to drive hospital practices today, with no signs of abatement.

Another arena of health care that participated in the opiate crisis is the role of the online pharmacy. While regulatory bodies now tightly control local pharmacies and the amount of painkillers they provide, including other medications that could potentially be made into drugs, online pharmacies have largely dodged this oversight. There are about 35,000 online pharmacies worldwide, and most are illegal. These online pharmacies can operate without regulation because their physical plants exist in foreign countries that don't monitor their practices. They don't need a prescription, and their medications are often unauthenticated. In many cases, overseas drug companies use these websites as a way to market their product to the consumer directly, avoiding the insurance middleman and pushing contaminated or faulty product. Even monitored websites have loopholes—those that allow for multiple accounts to be created and don't have an alert system for deliveries made to the same address. The profitability of online pharmacies has sparked the attention of one shipping giant, Amazon. Amazon intends to join the $400 billion pharmacy marketplace by acquiring PillPack Inc., an online pharmacy that targets chronically ill patients by packaging an entire month's worth of medication and delivering it to their home.

The marriage of Amazon to the prescription drug world only serves to illustrate how muddy the health-care waters have become. The new trend in health care is to have different segments of the field join forces. Health-care providers used to offer medical services. Insurance companies used to pay for those services for those with contracts. Pharmacies used to provide medicines on the order of health-care providers. All three entities were separate from each other, focusing on streamlining their own business and providing best practices. In recent years, however, acquisitions have become the norm. Insurance companies are buying health-care groups. Pharmacies are buying insurance companies. Tech companies are acquiring health-care devices. Hospitals are buying other hospitals. In a small subset of examples, CVS pharmacy bought Aetna insurance, Walgreens pharmacy bought Humana, UnitedHealth insurance bought health-care groups, and Kaiser Permanente combines all three. These mega-corporations serve to recreate the medical model into a profit machine. It's one reason why the opiate epidemic has been so difficult to eradicate—there is no incentive to fully solve the problem when billions are at stake and the biggest entities have their hands in all the pies.

The last piece to the growing opiate business is, paradoxically, the treatment programs set up to solve the opiate epidemic. Substance abuse treatment has evolved from the nonprofit arena, such as the original Betty Ford Clinic (founded in the early 1980s), into the current $35 billion enterprise. Entranced by the media saturation of drug addiction, entrepreneurs took note and set up pricey drug rehab programs aimed at the rich and famous. One such program is Passages, a luxurious 10-acre $15 million property situated on the Pacific oceanside, founded in 2001. It is the largest and most expensive program in Malibu, charging around $80,000 per month. Others followed suit, wooing celebrities to pay into their hefty price tags, offering amenities such as massages, private chefs, personal assistants, and spa treatments.

Then, in a boon to low-paid therapists looking to break into the industry, new measures set up by the Affordable Care Act of 2010 and the 2008 Parity Act made substance abuse treatment a necessary cost to insurance companies. Having guaranteed a payer source for Middle America, and without any real price tag parameters, rehab substance abuse programs popped up all along the California coast, and beyond. Insurance companies will pay over a thousand dollars a day for residential substance abuse treatment, and often five times that amount for residential detox. Since adults who are addicted may be unemployed and thus have a hard time obtaining insurance, most are forced to pay privately, only to find that real recovery is financially out of reach, circulating between prison and substandard care medical care. Specialized programs for teenagers carved a niche in the marketplace as well, aimed at parents bewildered by their child's substance abuse problem and willing to pay anything to resolve it, including high insurance copays and deductibles.

Do pricey residential rehab programs work? Studies evaluating the evidence claim that residential treatment programs can work, but cannot definitely claim that it works better than other types of treatment. More objective analysis needs to occur, but the secretive culture of addiction, due to pervasive stigmas against the illness and the nature of the illness itself, prevents any kind of objective analysis over sobriety outcomes. For example, Passages claims that their "cure rate" is 90%, although insiders confide that it's actually more like 10%. To boost their claim, they published a booked entitled *The Alcoholism and Addiction Cure*, generating millions more in profit. Many are critical of their methods, however, claiming that pandering to the egos of famous clientele became more important than data-proven treatment. Ever tongue-in-cheek, the notable gossip website Gawker said, "Looking at that roster, this place should just call itself 'Relapses.'"

The rehab industry suffers from a lack of regulatory oversight that implements best practices for resolving substance abuse issues. Instead, feel-good remedies and ideological sentiments override data-driven research. The primary treatment model is based on the 12-step program, first publicized by alcoholics as a cure for alcoholics in 1939. It's a series of steps based on religious belief in a higher power, created before neuroscience began real research into the area of addiction. Current peer-reviewed studies indicate that the success rate of the 12-step program is only about 10%, and yet the program is considered sacrosanct by its vocal proponents. In a society desperate to cure its mounting numbers of addicted people, many residential rehab facilities can deploy anything from belief in Jesus to horseback riding as a therapeutic program, and are able to market success rates that aren't verified by any third-party authentication sources. And surprisingly, many personnel assigned to treat the patients have little more credentials than a prior addiction themselves.

Most specialists trained in treating addiction state that one of the most important qualifications for sobriety in residential treatment homes is not just the therapeutic support, but also the amount of time spent in these places. Studies show that addicted people are more likely to maintain sobriety following a 90-day treatment program (minimum) versus programs that last much less. However, insurance companies are pushing back against their ACA requirements, setting caps well under a reasonable time frame for recovery, and encouraging more outpatient treatment instead. Responsible facilities that accept insurance payments are forced to step people down to a lower level of care before they are ready. Conversely, patients have accused private-pay facilities of deciding to discharge them to an outpatient facility coincidentally when the money finally runs out.

Outpatient substance abuse treatment is reimbursed at a considerably reduced rate than residential substance abuse treatment, which is why it's the preferred therapeutic model of insurance companies. However, outpatient treatment comes with pitfalls and flaws, much of it based on greed and lack of legal oversight. The main flaw of the outpatient model is that newly sober individuals are often forced to move back to their previous environment—a place that reminds them of times that they were high, a place that often contains the emotional triggers to drug use (such as volatile relationships with family and friends), and often puts them in close proximity to their former dealer.

To counter these problems, outpatient therapy is often coupled to sober living homes, in which a formerly addicted person will live drug-free amongst like-minded peers. Any house can be labeled a "sober living" home, and there are no caps on the amount of beds a sober living facility can provide, and currently no zoning laws against it. As people with substance addictions are considered handicapped under federal law, with all its inherent rights and protections, neighborhood residents have no recourse against the hundreds of sober living facilities cropping up around them. While this can help a newly sober patient maintain distance from his or her former life of using, it often backfires, with a constant barrage of reminiscing about days spent while high providing its own trigger to relapse. And, in a final blow to the recovering addicted, sober living rents are expensive.

Often, while insurance companies do not cover rent to stay in a sober living house, the outpatient facility (which often also own the home) will use a percentage of insurance reimbursements as a kickback to the facility for patient referrals, covering a portion of the rent. Most will even send a car to pick up patients from the sober living home to ensure compliance. Still others reward sober living residents with cell phones, gift cards, or other incentives to remain in their programs.

Another way sober livings and outpatient treatment centers have increased their income is by receiving kickbacks from urine tests. Urine tests are a necessary component of sober living, as a person who relapses is a threat to the sobriety of other residents. However, the frequency of urine tests became the focal point of an intense FBI investigation into the practice of urine testing, after Medicare, Medicaid, and therapists themselves felt duty bound to call attention to price gouging. Outpatient facilities and sober livings were testing patients seven days a week, charging patients and insurances thousands per sample. A typical urine test can cost around $25. Laboratories would offer kickbacks to facilities to use their services. Some owners of outpatient facilities and sober livings, seeing dollar signs, opened up their own labs to conduct urine analysis.

Private insurance took note and began suing facilities for fraudulent practices. In one example, Cigna sued Sky Technology for $20 million in civil fraud for offering drug treatment facilities ownership interests in their company that were dependent upon sending urine tests to Sky laboratories. While the actual dollar amounts are unknown, insiders say that doctors were paid up to $50,000 monthly for their continued patronage of their laboratories.

Other ways of patient brokering have emerged in a billion-dollar industry that's facing ever more competition. These include call centers that collect fees for patient referrals; "moles" that are hired to live in a sober living and lure others away to a different facility; cash payments to anyone who brings in users from the streets or the hospitals; and horrifyingly enough, even those who entice sober residents to relapse, so that they can get insurance companies to pay for the detox-residential-outpatient cycle all over again.

While legislation is emerging in states such as Florida, which was at the forefront of most of these unsavory practices, the problem is quickly becoming a national issue. And even after legislation has passed to make patient brokering illegal, cash payments cannot always be traced or proven, and evidence of wrongdoing is hard to come by. And finally, even with overwhelming evidence of misconduct, policing agencies are under-staffed and overwhelmed, and often lack real ways to exact penalties to the offenders.

In conclusion, the opioid epidemic began and is perpetuated by the very people involved in the business of our health. On every front, from the physician, to the pharmaceutical company, to the insurance, to the phar-macy, to the rehab centers, there is money to be made in the creation of an addicted individual and then treatment for the addiction itself. Profit from every avenue of health care created and perpetuated the opiate epi-demic. Discovering ways to incentivize optimal health, not simply the vol-ume of health care delivered, will be the only business model that leads us from this dark period in medical history to a brighter future.

CHAPTER 7

Harm Reduction

In the world of substance abuse, the concept of harm reduction has gained a great deal of momentum as study after study shows that it does not increase overall drug use or the number of people using drugs. The central principle of harm reduction is that even though drug use is not the best choice, steps should be taken to reduce negative consequences related to it. The National Harm Reduction Coalition writes, "Any reduction in harm is a step in the right direction." While harm reduction has always existed historically in some form, politically, it has generally been challenging to implement it. Fortunately, social activism and scientific advancement have made harm reduction available to many clinicians and their patients who are suffering with substance use disorders.

In the minds of many Americans, intoxication of any kind has always been shackled together with moral weakness. After all, President Ronald Reagan and his First Lady Nancy Reagan preached that all one needed to do was to "Just Say No" to drugs. While the message of their campaign against drugs can be seen as motivated by preventing the beginning of a harmful process, underlying it is the idea that anyone who has said "yes" is morally degenerate.

Also, during the 1980s, harm reduction would have been seen as being "weak on crime" and certainly would have been inconsistent with America's strong history of racial prejudice. The '80s War on Drugs, along with attacks on welfare, entwined poverty and drug use with being a problem confined to minority members. The result was an unhealthy soup of political apathy, spurning those who grew sick and died as "deserving" of their fate. Doing anything to reduce the harms of drug use would be helping those who are deserving of no help.

The crack cocaine epidemic of the 1980s illustrated just how political the issue had become. Crack cocaine use occurred mostly in the more poverty-stricken African American community. Alongside addiction came an increase in violence between drug dealers, between dealer and user, between rival gangs, and between the user and other members of family and community. This drug-related violence isolated and demonized the African American community. TV news filled Americans' living rooms with images of minority men suffering from crack addiction, serving to distance the majority of America from the problem. This distance served to further racist tendencies. Fearing further drug abuse and alienation of their community due to negative perceptions of the behavior, many leaders of minority communities supported harsh legal consequences for drug use. To date, many African Americans who use crack cocaine have a harder time accessing harm reduction programs due to sociocultural and socioeconomic factors.

A co-occuring crisis only weakly connected to crack use and far more connected to heroin may have paved the way for harm reduction in the United States. Activism and social justice intensified as a direct result of the skyrocketing rates of HIV in the United States. Until this point, most harm reduction was seen as aiding and abetting the behavior of a criminal. After the horror of AIDS patients was being telecast on the nightly news, the public became more willing to do whatever it took to stop the epidemic from entering their homes. While most didn't fully believe that substance abuse was a contagious disease, as scientists insisted, they nevertheless felt that harm reduction would be a necessity. These activist groups, such as the American Foundation for AIDS Research, were willing to fund harm reduction projects that mimicked programs from Amsterdam and the United Kingdom, rather than wait for taxpayer funds. This fast-tracked programs directly to the public, where their effectiveness could be measured.

Once doctors began to connect the dots between substance abuse and HIV infection, researchers felt it prudent to prevent drug abusers from sharing needles. This led to the growth of similar programs with similar names and philosophies including needle and syringe programs (NSPs), syringe exchange programs (SEPs), and needle exchange programs (NEPs). The purpose was to provide clean needles and syringes, alcohol swabs and pads, and sterile water to people who are already using injection drugs. Boston, Massachusetts, and Tacoma, Washington, were some of the earliest cities to start syringe service programs after seeing falling HIV rates in a similar Amsterdam program. Amsterdam has one of the highest rates of intravenous drug use in the world, and yet nearly eliminated HIV infection rates from sharing needles.

Public opinion of syringe service programs unfortunately remains poor, as various bans in U.S. history to funding these programs attests. However, a study following 1,577 intravenous drug users over a two-year span in California shows that these programs do work. Other studies based out of New York showed similar success rates. Those with access to clean syringes were more likely to take advantage of the program and not reuse syringes, whereas those without access to these programs were more likely to share syringes with others. Importantly, the greater access to more syringes did not impact disposal of these syringes. Meaning, parks didn't suddenly become filled with used single-use syringes.

Despite the obvious success of these programs, federal funds were banned from these exchanges until Congress relented in 2016. Governor Mark Pence of Indiana, now Vice President of the United States, declared a state of emergency after a steep rise in new HIV infections in the state—all traced to intravenous drug users abusing opiate painkillers. While he previously believed that allowing needle exchange programs to be funded by federal monies was a tacit approval of drug abuse, real-world consequences of the opiate epidemic forced him to reconsider. As a compromise, needle exchange programs aim not just to reduce infectious disease transmission rates, but also to provide drug treatment program information to their participants. And they work, but they work only when they are easy to use, local, and do not put unnecessary restrictions and judgment on the user.

In addition to needle exchange programs, communities have adopted seemingly unrelated programs that emanate from a harm reduction philosophy. After it became apparent that many individuals with addiction were too scared to call 911, many states have adopted a new law. This law offers assurance for anyone calling 911 to report a drug-related medical emergency will not be arrested by police. While some feel that this allows drug dealers to get away, most are in full agreement that it's more important to potentially save someone from an overdose than to penalize anyone from attempting to help.

The above measures don't necessarily help the drug-addicted person overcome his addiction, but they do shield him from bearing the full brunt of negative consequences related to his illness. They provide him with time and prolonged good health and further the chance for recovery.

Specifically, for opioids, harm reduction has yielded the most evidence-based solutions to addiction, medication assisted therapy (MAT). Drugs like heroin, OxyContin, and fentanyl literally change the chemical structure of the brain. Medications likes buprenorphine and methadone can meet the chemically altered brain where it is at and allow the individual in recover from addiction to live a life free of it.

Before delving into the history of MAT it is essential to understand that it is not "trading one addiction for another." Medications that are prescribed and monitored by a physician, such as methadone and buprenorphine, are fulfilling a physical dependence that people who have abused opioids have developed over time. The prescribed medications, as part of an overall recovery program, allow people to live lives similar to, or in some cases even exceeding in quality, the lives before drugs entered the picture. Individuals in MAT are workers, parents, business owners, and community leaders.

MAT can run into a great deal of opposition. Many 12-step supporters who believe that abstinence is the only solution eschew the scientifically based gains offered by MAT. They argue that medication assistance only trains the addicted to function while on drugs, while not addressing the problem of drug reliance in everyday life. Many believe that drug addiction emerges from some kind of psychological trauma or untreated mental illness, and only by addressing these inherent drives can an addicted person fully return to normal life. It is important when faced with people who invoke 12-step programs (like AA and NA) as being opposed to the use of MAT that the guidebooks for these organizations believe that any medication that is taken as prescribed by a physician is not inconsistent with a drug-free life. Those who claim methadone and buprenorphine are inconsistent with 12-step programs have their facts wrong!

The opposition to MAT in some parts of the 12-step world has historical basis. The first 12-step program, AA, was started by two men suffering with alcoholism who wanted to help others with the same struggle. Millions and millions of people have recovered from alcoholism worldwide through AA, and 12-step programs for other ills developed on the belief that other behaviors could be changed through the same means. This is why today we have Gamblers Anonymous, Overeaters Anonymous, and Narcotics Anonymous.

Unfortunately, though, the brain's response to opioids appears to be more enduring than to other substances. The recovery models that worked for other problems have simply failed to show any evidence of helping with opioid addiction. Once the brain gets used to living with opioids, the withdrawal effects don't just last for a few days—they can last for months or even years. In fact, brain scans show that a brain needs over a full year to recover normal function after its dependency on opiates. This is one reason why relapse is so high—the brain is still needing opioids to function well. Knowing this danger, says experts, is key to understanding why medication assistance treatment is so vital. It lowers the withdrawal effects of both the body and the brain.

Methadone was first created in a German laboratory in 1937 as a way to re-create opium during a national shortage. Side effects tabled the drug, and it only regained scientific interest in the United States in the late 1940s as street anecdotal data suggested it could be a way to wean off opiate addiction. Methadone isn't a great analgesic—its effects are milder than heroin and morphine, and it has a great deal of side effects. While morphine might linger for about one to five hours, methadone can stay anywhere from 15 to 60. Methadone was first considered as a sobriety strategy for opiate users in 1965, although the term "harm reduction" didn't exist then. Users quickly developed a physical tolerance to methadone, and report feeling very few pleasurable feelings from the drug within a few short weeks. This is the "sweet spot" of methadone—the ability to stimulate brain synapses, but the inability to feel "high," and thus impede day-to-day activities. For many, it is this sweet spot that enables them to be functional and unimpeded by the disease of addiction. And the data illustrates this; compared to controls, those taking methadone were four times more likely to stay in treatment and had a third as many positive drug tests. Crime is reduced, infectious disease transmission is reduced, and treatment improves most outcomes.

Many in methadone treatment programs unfortunately have to contend with baffling legal restrictions and loopholes that curtail normal activities. Many can't accept jobs or living accommodations that put them too far from a methadone clinic, as methadone must be administered by medical personnel daily. Only about half of all private-sector facilities that treat drug addiction use MAT. And in those facilities, only one-third of those patients actually receive medication. That's a shocking statistic. Essentially only a minority of people seeking help for drug addiction get the most evidence-based treatment for it.

Methadone clinics by law have to impose many restrictions on patients seeking care from them. Many patients report an ongoing power struggle to receive methadone. Because methadone is an opiate, because it has potential for abuse, and because when mixed with other drugs it can be dangerous, clinics impose a hierarchal order on who is able to receive the drug on a daily basis at first. This is motivated by the desire to block methadone diversion and to block people from getting a potentially lethal dose by taking more than one day's dose. Methadone must be administered in person, in liquid form, with mouth checks to ensure consumption. A urine test that shows the presence of other drugs and alcohol results may lead to restriction in privileges patient have—such as getting to take home several doses a day at one time.

In addition to methadone, Suboxone is another opioid that is used in MAT. It's considered less dangerous than methadone—methadone is a Schedule II drug, meaning it's highly addictive, and Suboxone is Schedule III, which is less addictive. To compare, Vicodin is also a Schedule III drug. Heroin is a Schedule I drug, considered too dangerous to ever prescribe and with no clinically valid purpose. Suboxone can cause similar side effects to methadone, including gastrointestinal issues and heart palpitations, but can be taken at home instead of a clinic.

The reason buprenorphine can be taken in the home has to do with the very nature of the drug molecule. Unlike methadone, buprenorphine cannot fully turn on receptors for opioids in the brain. When buprenorphine binds to the opioid receptor, it is like turning on a light but only to a dim level. This is known as a "partial agonist," and this partial agonist means that there is very little risk of fatal overdose. Continuing the simile from above, it also means that after you take enough of it the light cannot be turned on any brighter—it simply shines at a dim level. This means there is no motivation to take more than is prescribed.

Federal guidelines for physicians prescribing Suboxone have led to suboptimal availability of this medications. Physicians are limited in the amounts of patients they can prescribe, and they must receive special training. This limits resources for addicted persons searching for a physician to assist with MAT. Many physicians who are able to prescribe Suboxone have long waiting lists of patients who wish to see them but can't get in.

There is one medication-assisted therapy that is not based on opioid replacement but rather on blocking the effects of opioids. Naltrexone can be prescribed by any health professional with no limitations. It is injected monthly and has no potential for abuse. It works by combating the effects of the opioid. In other words, it eliminates any pleasure from taking heroin or other opiates, making the point in taking the drug obsolete. It also reduces cravings for the drug. There are several problems with naltrexone, however. One is that it is far more expensive than methadone and Suboxone, which limits its availability to those with good health insurance. Most limiting, it also requires the addicted to be opioid free for a period of time before beginning a regimen of the naltrexone. This is to avoid hurtling a drug-addicted person into immediate withdrawal upon taking the drug.

To combat illness felt during opiate withdrawal, doctors are implementing drugs aimed at lessening symptoms. Drugs such as Lucemya (lofexidine hypochloride), clonidine, guanfacine, and tizanidine are known as alpha-2-adrenergic agonists. They're most commonly used for high blood pressure and anxiety, which is often a symptom of withdrawal. In addition, they provide slight sedation to help users get through the worst of the withdrawal process. These withdrawal agents do nothing to prevent long-term drug abuse and should only be used as a bridge to naltrexone as opposed to an end goal.

Harm reduction with medication is not only for treating people with addiction to prevent relapse, but it can be to acutely save someone's life who has overdosed. Naloxone, popularly known as Narcan, is a medication that is an opioid antagonist, much like naltrexone but far faster acting. It works by countering the effects of the opioid. One of the side effects of opioids—indeed, the major cause of overdoses—is the fact that it has a sedating effect on the nervous system. It dampens the nerves, causes drowsiness, and affects breathing if taken in too high doses or combined with sedation-inducing drugs like alcohol, sleeping pills, and anti-anxiety medications. Narcan reverses the respiratory effects of an overdose. Narcan has been so instrumental in reversing a potential overdose that doctors are calling it a miracle drug. It is nonaddictive and works fast when injected. The results are so dramatic that Surgeon General Dr. Jerome Adams stated that "more Americans should carry and be trained to administer . . . Naloxone." Carrying Narcan might be a harm reduction strategy, but in this case, it's a nondisputed measure to an unfortunate trend.

Ultimately, none of the above MAT approaches have disadvantages, but they are perceived as having harms related to them. Despite decades of evidence of success, methadone remains controversial in the United States. Communities will often oppose the opening of methadone clinics in their neighborhoods despite the numerous neighbors who could be saved by these clinics.

The next idea is at the avant garde of harm reduction, and given America's uneasy relationship with harm reduction, it is difficult to imagine its implementation here. While methadone helps millions, some still cannot live lives free of heroin. For these individuals, Sweden took an unconventional and astonishing approach—medically prescribed heroin. They discovered that giving people who wanted to quit a syringe of heroin and a government space to do it in, alongside mandatory care programs, had far better results than controls or methadone treatment. Users were 23–25% more likely to stay in treatment than methadone patients. They also suffered far less side effects and were able to function in the workforce better. Heroin treatment also reduced use of other illegal drugs—a problem commonly found with methadone, which doesn't provide enough of a high to satisfy those trying to wean off of the drug, and therefore mix methadone with other drugs to maintain.

In keeping with accepted political policy, there are many who argue that abstinence is the only answer. But for a growing legion of neuroscientists, MAT is vital to solve the conundrum of drug addiction. According to various studies, the brain undergoes a radical change with each initial use of the drug. It conditions itself to rely on the heroin-induced rush of dopamine and cannot function without it otherwise. *The Lancet* published perhaps the most damning evidence of all. They took a small group of opioid-addicted people and assigned them to undergo either withdrawal and psychological treatment, or medically assisted treatment using methadone or Suboxone. At the end of one year, 20% of the first group were dead from an overdose, and no one stayed in treatment. In the second group, 75% were abstinent and all were still alive.

Harm reduction has been introduced to temper to ill effects of other drugs of abuse besides opioids. Mothers Against Drunk Driving (MADD) and Students Against Drunk Driving (SADD) do not seek to stop people from drinking, they just seek to reduce people from taking the potentially lethal step of drinking and driving. Reductions in drinking and driving have been stunning, and the low rate of traffic fatalities in the United States today can be directly tied to this reduction.

One very deadly drug class that has limited harm reduction methods developed around it are stimulants. Methamphetamine, a drug so heavily featured in the television show *Breaking Bad* it should have its own name in the credits, is one of the most alarming drugs on the street today. One dose can flood the brain with dopamine and deplete its reserves so heavily that the brain can be forever altered. The long-term abuse of "meth" can result in alarming side effects such as irreversible psychosis. It rewires the brain and causes brain cell death and damage, and brain recovery can be as long as 18 months. Everything about this drug is extreme, including the drug-seeking behavior.

Caregivers, doctors, and scientists are desperate to find the "methadone" to methamphetamine. Methadone currently does not help with meth addiction. In clinical studies are a host of drugs, such as antipsychotics like risperidone and even stimulants. The most promising, however, is using naltrexone to reduce the high that meth users would feel. In a UCLA-based study, meth users who were given naltrexone felt less effects of the drug and had less cravings for more. The difficulty is in getting recovering addicts to take it, because they know the point is to reduce the high. Enter the naltrexone implant. In theory, the implant would take the decision making out of the addicted person's hands and reduce drug use by reducing the cravings and the dopamine reward system in the brain. The problem lies with the drug delivery system, say doctors, because it would need to be a steady, consistent dose. However, when the implant works correctly, it can reduce relapse rates amongst opiate and methamphetamine-addicted individuals.

In the absence of MAT for crystal meth, harm reduction posters have attempted to mitigate the damage. Harm reduction includes reinforcing the need for safe sex practices. Counselors encourage avoiding alcohol, getting sleep, eating right, brushing teeth, and seeing a dentist. Drug counselors dealing with methamphetamine-addicted individuals are taught productive ways of dealing with psychosis and paranoia to relieve anxiety. Sadly, these harm reduction strategies do little to offset how destructive methamphetamine can be. There is no way to mitigate the brain damage other than encouraging users to stop taking the drug.

While many embrace the theory that a drug addiction is a disease and not a moral failing, the attitudes toward medication assistance treatment reveal that there are still many who oppose this philosophy. The false belief that individuals using MAT are unable to utilize the far superior "willpower" required to simply overcome any obstacles. In truth, an opiate-addicted individual entering a residential treatment center—one that does not differentiate between the different type of addictions, but rather applies a "one size fits all" approach—stands very little chance of lasting sobriety. Study after study regurgitates the finding that medication-assisted treatment, geared to the specific class of medication causing the patient harm, is the only way to recovery. Worse, rehab can actually harm addicted individuals who relapse by lowering their tolerance and making relapses fatal instead of simply unfortunate, because if they attempt to use the same high dose they used when they had high tolerance, this dose may be enough to cause overdose when they return to a state of low tolerance.

What is known beyond a shadow of a doubt is that harm reduction does not result in a worsening of drug problems. It allows people who are misusing drugs to stay safer until a time when a recovery can be made. To be against harm reduction now is to say that you either reject science or don't care to help those suffering from drug addiction.

CHAPTER 8

"Junkies" and "Addicts": Criminals in a War on Drugs or Casualties in an Opioid Epidemic?

As has been discussed at various points throughout this book, the nature of drug abuse involves complex interplay between the medical system and the criminal justice system. Taking a cultural-historical perspective, this chapter will explore in further detail the ways the U.S. government has attempted to combat drug abuse and prescription drug abuse throughout the years in order to better frame the ongoing debates on what should be the nation's drug policy.

RICHARD NIXON AND THE "WAR ON DRUGS"

Ever since the early 1970s, the efforts to stop the ill effects of drug abuse in the United States have been widely known as the "War on Drugs." The major strategies in the War on Drugs include harsher prison sentences for possession and dealing, crop eradication domestically and in foreign countries, anti-drug campaigns, policing of drug cartels by cooperation between American and international law enforcement agencies, tracking of controlled substances, and others. The term was first put forth by the administration of President Richard Nixon to describe his vision of a policy shift in how the government would approach drug addiction and illegal drug use. Nixon described drug abuse as "public enemy number one," and he argued for a pivot in the public imagination away from a notion of drug users as patients in need of treatment toward a view of them as criminals in need of law enforcement. An illuminating quote is found in an article that Nixon wrote in *Reader's Digest* in 1967 called "What Happened to America?" He said in regard to Detroit rioters that, "our opinion-makers have gone too far in promoting the doctrine that when the law is broken, society, not the criminal, is to blame." For decades, Americans have largely agreed with President Nixon. For example, in 1972 only 15% of Americans thought marijuana ought to be legal, compared to 86% who thought it ought to be illegal. U.S. drug policy has not switched course drastically since that time. Every president from Nixon through George W. Bush used the term War on Drugs to describe their drug policy. President Barack Obama (2008–2016) instructed his administration not to use this terminology, but President Donald Trump has since reintroduced it. President Trump has even gone so far as to suggest that drug dealers be given the death penalty.

Under Nixon's leadership, Congress passed the Comprehensive Drug Abuse Prevention and Control Act of 1970, also known as the Controlled Substances Act (CSA). The CSA introduced numerous major changes to federal drug policy. One of these major changes was that multiple existing federal agencies that dealt with drug abuse were centralized into one new law enforcement agency called the DEA (Drug Enforcement Administration), whose primary mission was and still is to combat illegal drug use and drug smuggling. The CSA also established a system to categorize drugs with abuse potential into five drug schedules, or lists, of controlled substances according to 1) whether or not the drug in question is determined to have abuse potential and 2) whether or not the drug is determined to have medical value. The law did not clearly define drug abuse, so it is the DEA that determines which drugs have high potential to be abused. Accepted medical use is determined by whether or not high-quality clinical trials exist documenting medical value. Drugs with high abuse potential and no accepted medical use (no high-quality clinical trials) are designated as "Schedule I drugs." These currently include heroin, LSD, marijuana, mescalin (peyote), MDMA, GHB, ecstasy, psilocybin, methaqualone (Quaalude), khat, bath salts (MDPV), and hundreds of other lesser-known compounds. For drugs that do have evidence of legitimate value in medical treatment, they are organized into Schedules II through V according to how high their abuse potential is. This act also established required strict regulation record-keeping by pharmaceutical companies and medical providers to track the drugs, and the restrictions on which drugs can be prescribed or used in research studies become increasingly strict as one moves from Schedule V toward Schedule I. This scenario creates a catch-22 for researching Schedule I drugs. The fact that these drugs are listed on Schedule I makes it difficult to get them approved for research studies and clinical trials, and yet the main reason they have been classified as Schedule I drugs in the first place is that no prior research exists on them.

BRIEF HISTORICAL PERSPECTIVES ON THE WAR ON DRUGS

The origins of the ideas behind War on Drugs and current drug policy are complex and varied. The following brief history provides a very broad and simplified account—by no means exhaustive—of some of the most influential historical antecedents and political movements in U.S. history illuminating the rationale for these policies.

The immediate historical context, just prior to Nixon's launching these policies, were the "culture wars" of the 1960s. In a way, the War on Drugs can be thought of as a political response to the perceived negative aspects of the radical societal changes occurring during this decade. Much of the current popular understanding of drug abuse and addiction stems from the culture wars of the 1960s. It is well known that a great deal of societal unrest occurred during this time. Dramatic cultural shifts occurred in response to the protest against the Vietnam War, the passing of the Civil Rights Act, the continued ascendance of feminism and women entering the workplace, the increased visibility of the hippie counterculture, and the increasing visibility of drug culture through psychedelic rock music and controversial public figures such as Harvard professor and scientist Tim Leary, who advocated widespread LSD use and for users to "turn on, tune in, and drop out" of mainstream culture. President John F. Kennedy was assassinated in 1963 at the beginning of the decade, and Dr. Martin Luther King Jr. was assassinated in 1968 at the end of the decade. Crimes of all types rose in America at the end of the 1960s and continued through the 1970s and 1980s before dropping precipitously in the 1990s through the present. The reasons why this rise in crime occurred from the 1960s through the 1980s, only to then to drop steadily in the 1990s, is still hotly debated. However, whatever the true causes for the increase in crime had been, the reigning theory in government policy of the time was that crime had increased because drug use had increased. This was not the first time that Americans had come out to fight forcefully against the social ills of intoxicants and addictive substances. Numerous efforts have been made throughout American history to curtail substance abuse.

The roots of the War on Drugs go back almost to the beginning of the United States itself. One of the earliest and most influential movements that attempted to combat addiction and intoxication occurred at the beginning of the nineteenth century. There was a social movement known as the Temperance movement that advocated against alcohol intoxication. During its initial phases, the movement mostly argued against use of hard liquor such as whisky or rum. Later, it moved toward advocacy of complete abstinence from intoxicants. These advocates of total abstinence from alcohol were called teetotalers. One of the earliest organizations related to the Temperance movement was the American Temperance Society, formed in Boston, Massachusetts, in 1826. Members of this group signed a pledge to abstain from alcohol, and meetings were held to discuss issues related to alcohol. By 1836, the group had over 1 million members and 2,200 chapters in different cities across the country. These membership numbers are especially impressive considering that the 1840 census counts the entire U.S. population at about 17 million total residents. There were numerous reasons for this swift growth. Religious fervor was high during these decades as the Protestant religious revival known as the Second Great Awakening attracted many members to Baptist, Methodist, and other church denominations who called for moral reform, including beliefs in the abolition of slavery as well as abstinence from alcohol. It is also important to note that this was largely a male phenomenon at the time. Men's alcohol consumption in the United States was much higher in those times. It is estimated the average man drank three times the amount of alcohol in the early nineteenth century as he does in the twenty-first century, and with increasing consumption of hard liquor, drunkenness became an increasing problem. For example, in Ken Burns's documentary *Prohibition*, in an interview with historian and author Catherine Gilbert Murdock, she says about alcohol use during that time period, "Alcohol consumption at that point was a sign of masculinity that took away masculinity, so that you drank to show that you were a man. But you get drunk, and all of a sudden you can't provide for your family, you can't do your job, you become violent. . . ." She notes that there was no divorce allowed at this time, and women did not have the right to vote. The gender-specific nature of this problem provided cause for women to band together as a group to fight for social change. Issues such as domestic abuse and marital rape, both of which were fueled by alcohol consumed by men at male-only saloons common at the time, could not be discussed in public. However, alcoholism itself could be addressed. Alcohol came to be seen as the cause of a great number of society's sins. These women who banded together into groups such as the Woman's Christian Temperance Movement and the Anti-Saloon League in the later nineteenth century to protest alcohol use soon discovered they had political power when they gathered in large numbers. The size and influence of these movements continued to grow through the early twentieth century, and prohibition of alcohol even became a rallying cry to mobilize women to fight for the general right for women to vote in order to gain to power to then vote for prohibition of alcohol. As the Temperance movement grew in influence through the end of the nineteenth century and the beginning of the twentieth century, total abstinence would prove a powerful stance on the issue of how to solve societal problems caused by addiction.

The culmination of the Temperance movement occurred in 1919 with the ratification of the Eighteenth Amendment to the U.S. Constitution, which prohibited the manufacture, transportation, and sale of intoxicating liquors and ushered in the era of Prohibition. (The Nineteenth Amendment, which gave women the right to vote, was ratified a year later.) Enforcement of Prohibition lasted until 1933 when the Twenty-First amendment was ratified, which repealed the Nineteenth amendment, ending Prohibition. By the time of repeal, many Americans had come to feel that the experiment had backfired. This was the era of bootleg liquor, gangsterism, Al Capone, and secret "speakeasy" bars that required a password to gain entry. It has since been widely recognized that Prohibition itself led to the formation of organized crime and an unregulated black market for the sale of unregulated alcohol. Similar to current street drugs, the alcohol sold on the black market during Prohibition was unregulated and contained harmful or even deadly impurities—for example, when methanol (wood alcohol) was mixed in with alcohol to stretch a supply. Large segments of the population—for example, many more recent European immigrants, often Catholics—did not share the puritanical view of total abstinence from alcohol that original settlers often held. This created an increasingly irreverent scofflaw attitude toward the government in which the general authority of the law was respected less. Despite the oft-noted failures of this era, it is fair to note that alcohol consumption did decrease in general, which caused large reductions in the number of cases of cirrhosis of the liver.

Another early historical precedent to the War on Drugs occurred in the in late nineteenth and early twentieth centuries when the general public as well as the medical establishment became increasingly aware of a growing epidemic of addictions to medications being prescribed by doctors. Particular concern surrounded cocaine, heroin, and morphine. Indeed, the current opioid crisis can be thought of as a second, successor opioid crisis with some parallels to the first. From colonial times until the early twentieth century, around the time of World War I, there were no federal laws restricting the sale of any drug in the United States. Prior to this, morphine, heroin, and cocaine were popularly used and prescribed medications. Some of the drugs that are highly regulated today were often available at that time without prescription. They were often sold in the form of patent medicines, which were commercially sold, name-brand medicines produced before the era of drug regulation that did not have to disclose their ingredients. They often purported to be made of special roots or herbs but in reality often contained substances such as opium or cocaine. The invention and increasing use of the hypodermic needle in the mid-nineteenth century also accelerated the incidence of addiction to injected morphine and cocaine, particularly among soldiers and veterans of the Civil War, as these instruments delivered doses more quickly and with greater potency.

As the addictive properties of drugs like morphine and cocaine became more apparent, and concerns about increasing use of intoxicants continued to rise, Congress passed the first act regulating the sale of opioids and cocaine, called the Harrison Narcotic Act of 1914, which restricted the sale of these substances to physicians and pharmacists using them for legitimate and professional practice. In the decades preceding the passage of this act, the United States had experienced what was essentially the country's *first* opioid crisis. While this law put more power in the hands of physicians and pharmacists to decide which medications a person could take, it also presented new liabilities to those providers. Prescriptions could be written only for legitimate medical practice. However, what constituted legitimate medical practice soon became hotly contested when physicians began prescribing these opioids to treat the physical dependency to help the addicted users avoid complications resulting from cessation (similar to the way methadone is used today). Soon, thousands of physicians, pharmacists, and patients involved in these treatments found themselves under arrest as law enforcement argued that such treatment was not legitimate medical practice. In 1919, the Supreme Court passed a ruling that was in agreement with law enforcement, and as a result, these physicians, pharmacists, and patients started to be put in jail. As a result, the prescription of opioids by physicians decreased dramatically for decades until increasing again in the late twentieth century when physicians began to feel increasingly concerned that patients' pain was not being adequately treated due to overly timid prescribing practices.

DEATH, VIOLENCE, AND THE WAR ON DRUGS

For many Americans, the idea of drug abuse is tightly wound with criminality and in particular, violent crime. For example, in a 2016 op-ed piece by Attorney General Jeff Sessions published in the *Washington Post*, he argues that the law enforcement policies toward "drug offenders" during the Obama administration were weak, and what was needed was a renewed tough-on-crime stance, including increased incarceration, in order to avoid an increase of violent crime. As he stated, "Drug trafficking is an inherently violent business. If you want to collect a drug debt, you can't, and don't, file a lawsuit in court. You collect it by the barrel of a gun. For the approximately 52,000 Americans who died of a drug overdose in 2015, drug trafficking was a deadly business." Following this, he pointed to a 2013 policy change at the Justice Department that decreased the number of federally imprisoned drug offenders by 23%. He then noted that violent crime had steadily decreased in America since the early 1990s, but that is had increased in 2015 by its largest amount in a single year since 1991.

While it is true that violent crime increased somewhat in 2016 as compared to 2015, it is notable that Mr. Sessions pointed to the drug overdose deaths as evidence of this increased violence. The mere fact that 52,000 people died from drug overdose deaths, while tragic, does not indicate that these deaths were the result of direct criminal violence. In fact, the largest portion of drug overdoses that year did not involve criminal drug deals at all. The majority of these deaths were not caused by black market drugs such as heroin and cocaine, but rather by prescription drugs of abuse such as prescription opioids. When the numbers are broken down, about 33,000 of those overdoses involved opioids. Of those opioid overdoses, about 17,000 involved prescription opioids, about 13,000 involved heroin, and about 3,000 involved synthetic opioids (predominantly fentanyl, much of it made illegally in China), making prescription opioids the number one source of overdose deaths that year involving opioids. Prescription benzodiazepines were involved in about 8,800 of the overdose deaths that year. As seen in previous chapters, prescription drugs of abuse are more commonly acquired through friends and family rather than from street dealers. Also noted in an earlier chapter, three out of four heroin users report having had an initial addiction to prescription pain medication before transitioning to heroin. Therefore, in pointing to the drug overdose death statistics that year as evidence of criminal drug violence, he seems to have confused drug-related violent crime with drug overdose deaths. Although criminal organizations that sell drugs, such as cartels or street gangs, are certainly social ills and partially responsible for the drug overdose epidemic, it is an oversimplification to solely blame criminal organizations for all the drug overdose deaths. Perhaps Sessions shared a view similar to Nancy Reagan, who argued for harsh prison sentences for drug possession. She was quoted in the late 1980s saying "if you're a casual drug user, you are an accomplice to murder." She was arguing that the money paid by the casual drug user then went on to fund criminal enterprise, which then resulted in deaths, for example, by violence between competing traffickers or by fatal overdoses of drugs sold by these traffickers.

According to the Bureau of Justice Statistics, violent crimes include murder, rape and sexual assault, robbery, and assault. In comparison to the drug overdose deaths, the homicide rate is actually much less. For example, the number of deaths as the result of physical violence (homicide, not drug overdose deaths) was a total of 17,250 homicides reported in the United States in 2016. The percentage of those homicides related to drug use or drug trafficking is difficult to quantify, since there are inconsistent definitions of what constitutes a drug-related crime, but the high estimate tends to be about 50% across studies. Of these, most are related to turf wars between traffickers. Perpetrators of violent crimes are more likely to be under the influence of alcohol than illegal drugs.

This violent crime rate has dropped consistently since the 1990s. The reasons for this are controversial and without expert consensus. However, it is interesting to note that the homicide rate in the 1970s and 1980s, following the implementation of the War on Drugs policies, reached levels previously seen only during the Prohibition era. It has been noted that the violent crime rate dropped significantly after Prohibition because organized crime crumbled when it no longer had a product as profitable as illicit alcohol to sell.

It must be noted that unlike violent crime, it has been shown that property crimes which include burglary, larceny, motor vehicle theft, and arson do increase as a result of increased drug use, because people with addiction can turn to theft as a method to get money to pay for their expensive drug habits.

INCARCERATION, RACISM, AND THE WAR ON DRUGS

The United States has the largest prison populations in the world, most of which are thought to be the result of harsh policies of the War on Drugs. According to the Bureau of Justice Statistics, in 2010 there were 2,266,800 people in local jails or in state or federal prisons, almost 1% of the total population of the United States. Many more are on probation or parole. In 2016, there were 6,613,500 people total under the supervision of the Department of Corrections, including local jail, state or federal prison, parole, or probation. The rate of incarceration has increased over 400% since the start of the War on Drugs. The rate of incarceration exploded after 1980, and many people point to mandatory sentencing laws of drug offenses as the reason for this. These laws were intended to deter drug use by imposing increasingly harsh minimum sentences for drug possession, often extending prison stays by years. For example, in the 1990s, the State of California introduced a "three strikes" law for drug possession in which a nonviolent offender who had three convictions for drug possession (e.g., greater than an ounce of marijuana) would be given a life sentence in jail.

Increased incarceration rates stemming from the policies of the War on Drugs have been criticized frequently. Blacks are overrepresented within the prison population as compared to their demographics in the nation as a whole. For example, a 2013 study conducted by the American Civil Liberties Union showed that though although blacks and whites use marijuana at similar rates, blacks are 3.73 times more likely to be arrested for marijuana possession. Given that there are about five times more white people than black people in the United States—and therefore five times as many white drug users as there are black drug users (since rates of use are similar)—many find it difficult to find an explanation for this discrepancy other than systemic racism. Political groups such as Black Lives Matter argue that unfair police practices targeting blacks explain part of this demographic discrepancy. It has also been frequently noted that mandatory sentencings laws starting in the 1990s unfairly targeted the black community—for example, by making possession of crack cocaine punishable by prison sentences up to five times longer than those for possession of powdered cocaine, crack cocaine use being historically more popular among blacks whereas powdered cocaine is historically more popular among whites. Although politicians supporting the War on Drugs would normally deny any racist agenda, an article written by journalist Dan Baum, published in the April 2016 issue of *Harper's* magazine, contained a quote from Nixon's former domestic-policy advisor, John Ehrlichman, that makes clear that a racist agenda was present within the policy from the beginning: "The Nixon campaign in 1968, and the Nixon White House after that, had two enemies: the antiwar left and black people. You understand what I'm saying? We knew we couldn't make it illegal to be either against the war or black, but by getting the public to associate the hippies with marijuana and blacks with heroin, and then criminalizing both heavily, we could disrupt those communities. We could arrest their leaders, raid their homes, break up their meetings, and vilify them night after night on the evening news. Did we know we were lying about the drugs? Of course we did." It has been noted that drug policies even in the early twentieth century often outlawed substances that were associated with minority ethnic groups. Opium dens in San Francisco were outlawed in the late 1800s and were associated with Chinese immigrants. Marijuana in the early twentieth century was associated with migrant Mexican farm workers. Cocaine and heroin gained associations with blacks in the early twentieth century as well, and stories about blacks becoming violent on cocaine were common among white people.

Privately owned prisons are another highly controversial phenomenon related to the increased incarceration rate associated with the War on Drugs. These prisons are run not by the government but by hired private contractors, typically for profit. In some cases, this has created a loop of corruption in which profits gained by these prison businesses have then been used to influence political figures in ways that increase profits further. For example, in 2011 a judge in Pennsylvania was himself sentenced to life in prison when he was found guilty of taking $1 million from a builder of for-profit prisons as part of a money-making scheme. In exchange for the money, the judge was found to have increased both the frequency of his guilty verdicts and the length of jail sentences that the guilty received. The purpose of this scheme was to increase the size of the prison population, which meant increased business for the company.

SHIFTING PUBLIC OPINION ON THE WAR ON DRUGS

Public perceptions about the War on Drugs have changed rapidly in recently years. For example, in 2013, for the first time in history, more Americans favored legalization of marijuana over continued criminalization. A nationally representative survey performed in 2014 showed that while 87% of people felt that drug abuse was either a "crisis" or a "serious problem," 67% of Americans now favored that the government take a more treatment-based approach to users of illegal drugs such as heroin or cocaine, while 26% preferred that such users be prosecuted (7% answered "don't know"). This included 51% of Republicans.

Public understanding of which drugs are the greatest threat seems to be shifting as well. In 2013, 63% of respondents said prescription drug abuse was an extremely or very serious public health problem. By 2018, the percentage had increased to 76%. By contrast, in 2018, two out of three Americans favored legalization of marijuana, including 51% of Republicans, the first time a majority of Republicans favored this policy. (Recall from earlier in this chapter that in 1971, 86% of Americans thought marijuana should be illegal.) Following the 2018 midterm elections, 10 states and Washington, D.C., had legalized recreational marijuana, and 33 states had legalized it for medical purposes. In the same year, America's close neighbor to the north, Canada, became the second country after Uruguay to legalize marijuana for recreational use. Canada has also legalized heroin for medical use in opioid maintenance therapy. Perhaps the increasing awareness of the role of prescription drug abuse in the nation's drug abuse problems is partly responsible for this shift in public opinion away from a criminal justice model toward a more treatment-based model, since prescription drug abuse is less associated with criminals.

At the time of writing this publication, there are signs that the political winds may be headed toward prison reform, and so greater leniency may soon take place. President Donald Trump, despite his past suggestions of the death penalty for drug dealers, has just publicly endorsed a prison reform act, currently called the Sentencing Reform and Corrections Act, which is being developed by Senate Republicans. Some of the proposals so far include decreasing the severity of penalties for low-level nonviolent drug offenses, increasing job and education training opportunities in prison, and removing minimum required sentences for drug offenses. The still Republican-controlled House of Representatives already passed their own version of the bill several months ago, and this passed with bipartisan support from both Democrats and Republicans. President Trump fired Jeff Sessions from his then-position of attorney general, and so the Justice Department will likely no longer pursue goals such as increasing the incarceration rate for drug-related crimes.

FRONTIERS IN DRUG POLICY

Since 2001, Portugal has followed a drug policy radically different than other countries when it passed a law decriminalizing consumption and possession of all illicit substances, as long as a person's supply is below established limits. (Drug dealing is still illegal.) This meant that people with addiction would no longer face prison for using, but instead would face at worst a warning, a fine, or a referral for services to treat their addiction, such as therapy or methadone maintenance. The result was not that the drug problem exploded, as some might have expected, but rather rates of drug-related harms of addiction, drug-related crime, overdose deaths, and transmission of HIV seem to have sharply fallen. For example, with opioid users able to come out of hiding, harm reduction methods such as needle exchanges could be utilized without fear of going to prison. In 2015, the nation's HIV infection rate dropped to 4.2 new cases per million people from the much higher rate of 104.2 new cases per million people in the year 2000. According to the Portuguese government, the total number of heroin users in the country has decreased to an estimated 25,000, down from 100,000 the year the law was enacted. The overdose death rate there dropped 85% over the same time period.

Some ideas similar to those in Portugal have taken hold in a handful of small towns in the United States. In 2015, the local police chief in the town of Gloucester, Massachusetts, decided to address a growing overdose death toll by announcing a new policy that anyone seeking help for opioid addiction could come to the police station and get a referral, without fear of arrest. The program has since expanded to hundreds of local police departments across the nation as of 2018 under the umbrella of a new organization called PAARI (Police Assisted Addiction and Recovery Initiative).

In addition to new ways of looking at addressing the social ills of drug addictions, a new look is also cautiously being taken at numerous illicit drugs currently listed as Schedule I, which by definition means they have no accepted medical use, and reevaluating them for any potential usefulness in medicine that was not previously appreciated. In earlier chapters it was noted that MDMA (Ecstasy) is currently beginning Phase III clinical trials for treatment of post-traumatic stress disorder by using it as an adjunct to assist psychotherapy and help people such as veterans to process and move on from past traumatic experiences. Researchers of psilocybin, the psychoactive drug found in hallucinogenic mushrooms, received approval from the FDA in November 2018 to perform clinical trials of this substance to treat refractory depression. Stigma within the scientific community toward serious research into these and other molecules such as psychedelics still exists, but it appears to be decreasing compared to prior years. Trials of many of these substances have not been performed for decades, even though the existence of these substances has been known for a long time.

As such research becomes more accepted, however, caution must be taken. As was noted to this writer in a discussion with the chair of our psychiatry department, Dr. Jonathan Alpert, there was much excitement in the 1970s and 1980s surrounding the increased use of opioid medications for the improved treatment of pain. He said contrary to what is often said in the media and otherwise, there was genuine idealism in the idea of improving treatment of pain and making patients' pain a greater priority. He then pointed out that despite these good intentions, the results may not be predictable. He said he is hopeful about the possibility of finding new chemical mechanisms and new possibilities of drug development by researching some of these currently illicit Schedule I drugs, but at the same time, the medical community must remain cautious that they do not inadvertently set off another wave of prescription drug abuse.

Another major risk involved in easing drug policies would be increased use among youth. The human brain continues to develop throughout adolescence and even into early adulthood. Psychoactive substances used during these life stages can potentially affect brain development negatively and increase the likelihood of addiction later in life. Continued education about the risks of using these substances for youth, as well as prohibiting use and purchase of many of these substances until a certain age, just as buying alcohol is prohibited until age 21, would likely be required.

The complexities of drug policy and the public's views on substance use ensure no easy solutions will be found to the problems created by substances with potential for abuse. Lloyd Sederer, MD, in his book *The Addiction Solution*, offers what is perhaps a good place to start reframing what the problem of drug abuse actually represents: "The metaphor the War on Drugs presupposes an enemy outside our borders or a civil uprising threatening the future of the nation. This is where the metaphor—applied to drugs as well as poverty and cancer—fails us from the very start. There is no external enemy. Drugs are what people with addictions use. They are not armies at the gate."

PART III

Scenarios

Case Studies

The following cases are drawn from elements of real patients and written to illustrate how different choices made by individuals interact with different systems in ways that contribute to the complex phenomenon of prescription drug abuse.

Case 1

Jenna is a 19-year-old female, white, upper-middle-class college student with ADHD at the University of Texas in Austin. She just started her sophomore year, and she recently started taking Adderall (mixed amphetamine salts) again after having attempted to wean herself off the medications during the second semester of her freshman year. She had always resented taking the medications when she was younger, feeling she was being forced by her parents and teachers to take medication she didn't want to take. She felt she had learned the coping skills she needed to succeed without the medications and felt that she was old enough now to no longer need them, since many children with ADHD find that their symptoms go away as they get older. However, her attempts to wean herself from the medication were not as successful as she had hoped. While she had earned A's and B's in her classes during her fall semester freshman year, she found that her grades dropped to mostly C's during her spring semester. She also noticed she was much less organized at home, leaving piles of papers around her room and letting all the household chores go unfinished. Her roommates began complaining that she wasn't doing her fair share and that she was becoming "lazy." She began forgetting plans she had made with her friends and was increasingly described as being more "flaky." She became concerned that her inattentiveness and disorganization were affecting her relationships with her roommates. Additionally, she desired to go to law school after finishing her undergraduate studies, and so she became concerned that stopping her ADHD medications would jeopardize her future plans, so she decided to restart her ADHD medications. She became rededicated to her career path to be a lawyer and determined to do whatever she needed to do to conquer her symptoms. In addition to medications, she went back into therapy, working to increase her organizational skills and also learning CBT (cognitive behavioral therapy) and mindfulness techniques to train her mind to focus better. She became friends with other like-minded, academically oriented peers and formed a study group. Her grades in the fall semester of her sophomore year greatly improved to mostly A's.

Analysis

In this case, Jenna uses Adderall, a controlled substance with high abuse potential, to help her focus on her studies. She uses the medication as prescribed, for treatment of her ADHD. During the time when she stopped using it, she noticed her functioning at school and her relationship with her roommates were suffering. She came to a new appreciation for the ways the medication helped her to maintain healthy work and interpersonal behaviors. Therefore, her use in the previous paragraph could not be categorized as prescription drug abuse. Her case illustrates the benefits and importance of having these controlled substances available for patients despite the risks involved in doing so.

CASE 2

Chad, a 19-year-old white male student, is a friend of Jenna (from case 1). He recently tried Adderall for the first time, which he obtained from Jenna. As the semester progressed, Jenna found she had more ADHD medication than she needed to do well, because she didn't take the medication every day as the psychiatrist prescribed (e.g., on the weekends). Since her study group friends were as academically inclined as she was, she began doing her friends a "favor" by sharing some of her ADHD medication with them. Her friends gladly accepted since ADHD medications help improve peoples' focus even for those who don't have ADHD.

Her friends study together with her and find the medication helps them achieve better grades in shorter time due to their increased focus. They became increasingly fond of the medication. One day, Chad asked Jenna for some Adderall to help study, but Jenna informed him she didn't have enough to spare for the month since much had been used already. Chad then checked a message board on a social media group related to his college, and he found another student offering to sell his Adderall for $10 a pill. Chad bought three 20mg pills. He used two for studying and saved the other one for an upcoming house party, since taking Adderall during a party could help him stay up all night. After arriving to the house party, he took one 20mg pill at 10pm, and another at 1am. Throughout the course of the evening, Chad proceeded to drink copious amounts of lager beers. He does not realize it, but the stimulant effects of the Adderall can often mask the feeling of being drunk. Users can feel as though they are not drunk despite having objective losses in judgment and difficulty with balance. As a result, he did not realize how inebriated he was becoming. Around 3:00am, two of his friends told him they were ready to go home and asked him to drive. Although he had drunk 10 beers over the past five hours, Chad felt he was sober enough to drive, and so he agreed. They passed him the keys, and an inebriated Chad took the wheel.

Analysis

This case is an example of a "diversion" of a prescription drug, because although Jenna obtained the drug legally, she illegally gave it away to her friends. Jenna did not actually abuse the drug herself. She initially saw her giving the Adderall away to her friends as a way to help them improve their grades—that is, she was passing them the drug to use as a performance enhancer. She may have felt it was not a big deal and may not have seen the consequences beyond the immediate effects that her friends felt on the drug while in their study session. Many misused prescription drugs are acquired in this way, which is almost impossible for police to detect. Indeed, Jenna and her friends may not have considered themselves to be doing anything particularly wrong or illegal. Her friends likely did not equate illegally taking her prescription ADHD medication as equivalent to taking an illegal drug such as heroin, cocaine, or marijuana. Nonetheless, she was giving powerful stimulant medication to her friends that could have consequences as dangerous as consequences from any of those drugs. Her enabling of her friends to try this medication seeded Chad's interest in it. This resulted in his escalating misuse of Adderall as a party drug, using it not to study but rather to increase his ability to remain awake and sociable during a party. He mixed the Adderall with another substance of abuse as well, alcohol. He was not aware of the way Adderall's effects mask the feeling of drunkenness. As a result, he underestimated how intoxicated he was, and he agreed to drive two other drunk friends, despite having drunk 10 lager beers himself that evening. In this way, Adderall contributed to his putting his friends' lives at risk by impairing his judgment and contributing to his decision to drive drunk. As for Jenna and others who are giving away or selling their ADHD medications, despite not being directly responsible for Chad's choice to drink and drive, it is important to note that those who divert medications still play a role in a larger systems issue by which powerful controlled substances are distributed to nonpatients and for nonprescription purposes.

CASE 3

Carlos, a 42-year-old male, Hispanic army veteran living in the Bronx, New York, has post-traumatic stress disorder (PTSD) after witnessing his best friend die violently in combat. He is divorced and has two sons who live with their mother. Ever since returning from the wars in Iraq and Afghanistan, he has had trouble identifying and interacting with civilians, and he spends much of his time alone living in an apartment paid for with public assistance. As part of his PTSD, he suffers from numerous psychiatric symptoms that are very debilitating to him. On an average day, he would describe his mood as either "numb" or a combination of anxiety, anger, and depression. He has hypervigilance, meaning he is perpetually easily startled and on the lookout for danger, as though enemy combatants might be waiting around any corner. He is afraid to leave his apartment unless it is absolutely necessary. He is afraid that he may be attacked by criminals living in the neighborhood, and likewise he is afraid that he may react explosively to any perceived threat. He has frequent flashbacks to his time in war, and he has frequent nightmares about combat when he tries to sleep. Eleven years ago, in order to treat his anxiety symptoms, one of his former doctors at the VA (hospital run by the Department of Veterans Affairs) had prescribed him Xanax for panic symptoms. Eventually, his dose was increased and he was taking Xanax multiple times per day. He never felt it helped his symptoms very much, but it was better than frequently leaving his apartment to go to weekly therapy sessions. Four years ago, when he discovered that people he knew would pay him large amounts of money to sell them his Xanax, he weaned himself slowly off the drug in order to sell it. The original doctor who prescribed Xanax to Carlos had left the VA many years ago, but Carlos had a new psychiatrist at the VA, Dr. Park, who has continued to fill his Xanax prescriptions. Even though Dr. Park is not the original doctor who initially prescribed Xanax to Carlos, she continues to prescribe it to him because Carlos is still clearly anxious, he still endures panic attacks, and he claims to continue to take Xanax as prescribed. As a result, Dr. Park concludes he has benzodiazepine dependence and would withdraw without his Xanax. As far as she knows, he takes it as prescribed. Each month, Carlos sells his entire bottle of Xanax to his friend Rafael in order to generate extra income. The ability to make extra income in this way is very important to Carlos because, having a debilitating disability such as severe PTSD, he feels he has few ways he is able to make extra money in the world and provide for his children.

Analysis

Carlos's case exemplifies many systems issues that allow for diversion to occur. He was prescribed Xanax years ago, and his doctors feel obliged to keep prescribing it, since he would withdraw without it (if he were actually taking it). This case is also an example of changing practice guidelines through the years creating problems. Carlos is clearly continuing to suffer due to his real PTSD symptoms as a result of witnessing the death of a friend in combat (and likely only nearly escaping death himself). He is continually on edge and finds it hard to integrate back into civilian life. According to the National Center for PTSD, about 8% of veterans in the United States suffer from PTSD. However, Carlos finds it a struggle to leave his apartment as a result of the PTSD symptoms, even to get the therapy which is ultimately needed to help his disorder improve. He finds that the benzodiazepine Xanax has not helped alleviate his symptoms of panic as much as he would like, and therefore he decides he would get more benefit from selling the medications to a friend. Xanax often sells on the street for about $2 per milligram, and it would not be uncommon for a person to be prescribed 3mg per day. Over the course of 30 days in a month, this means one bottle could sell for $180. Even if Carlos sells this bottle to Rafael for $100, an extra $100 a month for an unemployed person on disability can be a lot of money. Unlike Jenna in the previous example, who thinks she is merely giving prescription drugs to her friend to help him study, Carlos here is knowingly selling to an established drug dealer. He may feel it is worth telling a lie to his physician in order to get money to provide more funds to his children, since he may feel he has no other option to get extra funds due to his mental illness. The psychiatrist in this scenario, Dr. Park, has been put into a situation where she is prescribing benzodiazepines to a patient who has legitimate anxiety symptoms but who, unbeknownst to her, is not using the medication to treat his legitimate psychiatric illness. She can recommend other, more appropriate treatments for PTSD, such as an antidepressant and weekly talk therapy sessions, but if he disagrees, she cannot force him to switch to another medication and go to therapy sessions. Charged with caring for a patient in a public system who is otherwise non-adherent to recommended treatment, she may feel that keeping him on Xanax is the least harmful option she has, since she thinks he may go into a deadly withdrawal syndrome without the benzos. For these many reasons, Carlos still gets a prescription of Xanax after all these years, even though he does not take the drug.

CASE 4

Rafael, a 41-year-old male, Hispanic army veteran also living in the Bronx, New York, has known Carlos for several years. Though he was a veteran, Rafael found it difficult to adapt to the civilian workforce, and to make money he began selling drugs of several types, including prescription drugs and heroin. After receiving the full bottle of Xanax from Carlos, Rafael offered to sell some to two of his regular clients, Rocco and William, two other veterans he knows who also suffer from mental illness but who also have substance abuse problems, live in a homeless shelter, and use heroin. He also sold them several bags of heroin. That evening, Rocco and William went to hang out at a friend's apartment in the Tremont neighborhood. Everyone at the apartment was getting high on heroin, Xanax, and beer. As the hours ticked by, Rocco and William became increasingly intoxicated and sleepy, and they both passed out on the couch at their friend's apartment. The next morning, William was unable to wake Rocco from his sleep. He called 911. When the paramedics arrived, Rocco was found to be unresponsive, not breathing, and without a pulse. The autopsy report shows that at the time of his death, his blood tested positive for benzodiazepines, alcohol, heroin, and fentanyl. Fentanyl is a prescription opioid similar to heroin but much more potent. It is frequently mixed with street heroin to help maximize profits. Rocco's cause of death was determined to be an overdose caused by a combination of all four of the intoxicants he was taking at that time. Benzodiazepines and opioids decrease the body's respiratory drive, and so with so many of these drugs in his system, he simply stopped breathing.

Analysis

Even though Carlos and Dr. Park feel they are doing the best they can in a situation, the downstream effect is that Carlos's selling his Xanax has resulted in the death of a drug user, as the combination of opioids with benzodiazepines can result in accidental overdose. To make matters worse, Rafael sold heroin to Rocco and William that was apparently laced with fentanyl, a prescription opioid that is 50 times stronger than heroin and is sometimes used to help stretch out a heroin supply. Heroin dealers do not often know how to precisely convert heroin dosing to fentanyl dosing, and as a result, it is not uncommon for a bag of heroin cut with fentanyl to have a much greater potency than the user expects, resulting in accidental overdose.

CASE 5

Gladys is a 71-year-old African American female living in Cleveland, Ohio. She worked for many years as a public school teacher and is still considered a community leader by her friends, family, and fellow churchgoers. She has been happily married over 50 years. She has two sons and two daughters, and she has 10 grandchildren. She is highly respected by her family as a source of strength and positivity, and they frequently look to her for support and leadership, just as they have for decades. Occasionally she helps out with her children's' finances if they run into trouble, but they always pay her back. She remains active in the lives of her children, continues to have an active church life, and maintains an active social life among peers her own age. Despite her continued active lifestyle, she has developed several painful medical conditions as she has grown older, and as a result, she has been prescribed increasingly larger doses of pain medications over the past 20 years. She walks with the aid of a walker. She has a herniated disc between two of her lumbar vertebrae that push into her spinal cord and cause shooting pains down the back of her right leg where her sciatic nerve is located. For years she has had worsening osteoarthritis in multiple joints, including knees, hips, and spine. She is obese and suffers from low back pain. To help with her pain, she has been maintained on 10mg oxycodone four times per day, plus an additional "as needed" doses of 5mg oxycodone three times per day for "breakthrough pain." Over the years, she has developed tolerance to pain medications and has required increasingly high doses. She also takes Flexeril (cyclobenzaprine) 10mg three times per day for muscle spasms in her low back. Gladys considers herself a devout Christian, and as part of her religious upbringing, she has always eschewed alcohol, cigarettes, or any illegal drug, as she considers intoxicants such as these to be pollutants to her body, which she considers God's temple. About two years ago, she had a total knee replacement surgery in her left knee, and she was given additional pain medications at that time to cover the pain caused by the knee surgery that was in addition to her existing pains elsewhere in her body. The surgeon only gave her enough additional pain medication to cover her during the weeks following her surgery, but after this she was lowered back down to her regular pain medication dosages like she had pre-surgery. The pains in her hip and back joints were worse than before the surgery. She felt like her pain was not being adequately covered after the surgery, and she became increasingly desperate. The pain medication doctor did not want to raise her medication regimen because he was concerned she was becoming addicted. She was referred to a pain specialist, who prescribed her some non-opioid pain medications for pain, but again she felt her pain was not being adequately covered. As a result, she suffered.

Analysis

Gladys is certainly physically dependent on opioid pain medications considering how long she has been taking them, as evidenced by the fact that she has gained a tolerance to them through the years. The doctor and patient here are left in a difficult situation whereby the patient, who is already on long-term opioid treatment for years, is asking for increased doses. Given the current opioid epidemic, where tens of thousands of people are dying from prescription opioid overdoses, the pain doctor is likely concerned about enabling the addiction of a patient and may be wary to increase doses. However, this does not mean the patient is not legitimately having increased pain, even intolerable pain. The patient's chronic pain will not be well treated by additional opioid medications, because it is not likely to ever completely resolve. The patient likely does not think of herself as addicted, as she has always stayed away from intoxicants. However, it is possible for someone to go her whole life sober, only to become addicted to prescription drugs later in life. Some men or women in her situation, even such a high-standing, respected women as Gladys, have been known to uncharacteristically buy illegal prescription opioid drugs from street dealers when they feel they cannot get their pain treated adequately by their physician. Some otherwise lawful citizens in this situation have even been known to progress to heroin, since it is an opioid medication as well and can sometimes be cheaper than buying prescription painkillers from a pharmacy.

TIMELINE

The following is a brief timeline of some key events in the history of prescription drug abuse, as pertains to the United States.

1803   Morphine first isolated from opium poppy by Friedrich Serturner

1827   Beginning of commercial production and sale of morphine by the company that eventually became the modern pharmaceutical company Merck

1850s   Widespread sale of unregulated patent medicines takes hold in United States. At this time, there is no federal regulation requiring safety testing or appropriate labeling of ingredients in medications.

1860   German chemist Albert Niemann describes the isolation of pure cocaine from the coca leaf.

1861   Start of the American Civil War. Morphine was used extensively by wounded soldiers. Hypodermic syringes, which allowed faster and more potent drug delivery, were developed around this time, and their use became more popular as designs improved.

1864   Barbituric acid, a precursor to barbiturates, is discovered by a German chemist named Adolf von Baeyer.

1874   Diacetyl morphine (heroin) first synthesized in British chemist C. R. Alder Wright

1887   Japanese chemist Nagai Nagayoshi first isolates the chemical ephedrine from ma-huang.

1887   German scientist Lazar Edethe first synthesizes the amphetamine molecule.

1893   Japanese chemist Nagai Nagayoshi first synthesizes methamphetamine.

1898   Bayer company begins branding and selling the drug diacetylmorphine under the name "heroin" for its purported heroic qualities.

1903   Two scientists at the Bayer pharmaceutical company, Emil Fischer and Joseph von Mering, synthesize a chemical related to barbituric acid called barbital that helps relieve anxiety and insomnia, giving rise to the barbiturate drug class.

1906   Pure Food and Drug Act is passed. Products containing narcotics (patent medicines) now required to print this on label. The passage of this act was greatly influenced by the book *The Jungle* by Upton Sinclair.

1913   Bayer stops production of heroin due to reports of growing heroin related hospital admissions.

1914   Harrison Narcotic Act is passed, the first federal law in the United States to regulate the production and sale of narcotics such as opiates and coca products.

1924   Heroin is completely outlawed.

1937   Congress passes the Marihuana Tax Act, taxing the sale of marijuana or hemp.

1937   The synthetic opioid methadone is developed by German scientists to address a shortage of natural opioids.

1937   Elixir sulfanilamide tragedy occurs in United States in which hundreds of people die from poisoning from improperly prepared medication. This elixir was made by dissolving the antibacterial medication sulfanilamide into a solvent called diethylene glycol, which is poisonous. The pharmaceutical manufacturers, S. E. Massengill Company, did not test the elixir for safety, and they were negligent in that studies had already been published that described the toxic nature of this solvent. Public outrage related to this tragedy resulted in Congress passing the Federal Food, Drug, and Cosmetic Act the next year.

1938   Congress passes the Federal Food, Drug, and Cosmetic Act (FFDCA), which gives the Food and Drug Administration (FDA) authority to regulate the safety of drugs, medical devices, cosmetics, and food.

1956   Narcotics Control Act passes, allowing for the death penalty for the sale of heroin to a child by an adult.

1957   The first benzodiazepine to be synthesized, chlordiazepoxide (Librium), is developed by chemist Leo Sternbach while working at the Hoffmann-La Roche pharmaceutical company.

1959   Fentanyl, a highly potent opioid, is developed by Paul Janssen of Janssen Pharmaceutical.

1966   The Narcotics Rehabilitation Act passes, allowing court-mandated addiction treatment.

1969   A study conducted by psychiatrist Dr. Robert DuPont shows an association between crime and heroin addiction in that 44% of new inmates entering the Washington, D.C., jail tested positive for heroin on a urine drug test. This study gives a rationale for allowing the establishment of methadone clinics for treatment of heroin addiction.

1969   President Richard Nixon calls for a new national antidrug policy and describes drug abuse as a "serious national threat."

1970   Comprehensive Drug Abuse Prevention and Control Act is passed, leading to controlled drug schedule system.

1971   President Nixon declares a "war on drugs."

1973   Drug Enforcement Administration (DEA) is founded.

1986   Anti-Drug Abuse Act of 1986 is signed by President Ronald Reagan, creating mandatory minimum sentences for drug offenses. This law has been criticized for establishing longer prison sentences for crack cocaine, more often used by black Americans, than for powder cocaine, more often used by white Americans.

1990s   First wave of increased opioid overdose deaths in the current opioid epidemic. This wave occurred mostly as a result of increased abuse of prescription opioids (mostly natural opioids, semisynthetic opioids, and methadone). This coincides with the increased prescription of opioid pain medications by physicians, who were attempting to address a perceived undertreatment of pain and underuse of opioids for pain.

1993   North American Free Trade Agreement is signed by President Bill Clinton. The increase in legal trade and traffic across the U.S.-Mexican border allowed for increased smuggling of narcotics in the United States.

1995   FDA approval obtained for OxyContin, the long-acting version of the semisynthetic opioid oxycodone. It was believed at this time that OxyContin was less addictive than previously available prescription opioid medications.

1996   American Pain Society recommends idea of "Pain as the 5th Vital Sign" as part of a campaign to increase the treatment of pain among all patients. The traditional four vital signs that physicians check on every patient are the heart rate, blood pressure, temperature, and respiratory rate.

1996   The Comprehensive Methamphetamine Control Act is passed by Congress, increasing restrictions and penalties for possessing chemicals and equipment used in the manufacture of illicit methamphetamine.

2002   Turning point for prescription drug overdose deaths in the United States: every year since 2002, the number of overdose deaths involving prescription opioids has surpassed the number of overdose deaths involving heroin.

2009   Prescription drug abuse–related visits to emergency departments reach about 1.2 million cases, an increase of about 98% since 2004. Most of these visits were related to opioid pain relievers.

2009   The Drug Enforcement Agency cites prescription drug abuse as the nation's primary drug abuse problem.

2010   Second wave of increased opioid overdose deaths begins. This period of rapid overdose increase was mainly attributable to increased use of heroin.

2010   Congress passes the Fair Sentencing Act (FSA), which decreases the penalties tied to crack cocaine offenses to be more equal to the penalties given for powder cocaine offenses.

2013   Third wave of increased opioid overdose deaths begins, mostly attributable to increased use of illicitly manufactured fentanyl (IMF) and other synthetic opioids found mixed in with heroin, counterfeit prescription pills, and cocaine

2015   FDA approves intranasal naloxone, an opioid overdose antidote in the form of an easy-to-use nasal spray that can be administered by nonmedical professionals in emergency situations.

2017   Number of drug overdose deaths in the United States rises to over 70,000 per year, a mortality rate that is over six times greater than in 1999. Opioids account for 68% of these deaths (including legal prescription opioids as well as illegally produced opioids). Between 1999 and 2017, over 700,000 Americans died from drug overdose.

Acute pain: Pain that has a relatively quick onset and usually resolves in less than a month.

Addiction: A disease of strong and habitual want that causes a person to have significantly less self-control and as a result leads to moral failings and harmful behaviors.

Adverse childhood experiences (ACEs) Traumatic or stressful events experienced during childhood such as abuse or neglect

Amphetamines Class of stimulant drugs consisting of molecules derived from ephedrine, a naturally occurring stimulant molecule found in the *ephedra sinica* plant species

Analgesic Medicine with pain-relieving properties

Anesthetic That which causes insensitivity to pain

Antipsychotic Drug class functioning primarily to block D_2 dopamine receptors in the brain and decreasing many of the symptoms of psychosis, such as auditory hallucinations, delusions, or disorganized thoughts

Anxiety One of the primary emotions, characterized by fear and nervousness

Anxiety disorders Category of mental illnesses characterized by overactive anxiety responses in the body that are severe enough to impair one's ability to function in domains such as school, work, or social settings

Anxiolytics see **sedative-hypnotics**

Automatic behavior Behavior that occurs often out of conscious awareness as a result of encountering a stimulus; for example, a smoker could develop an automatic behavior when stress or anxiety causes him or her to light up a cigarette with very little conscious thought about whether or not to do so.

Benzodiazepines Class of CNS depressant drugs that slow down the rate of neural transmission in the brain by increasing the release of the GABA neurotransmitter

Bipolar disorder Mood disorder characterized by episodes of highly elevated mood (mania or hypomania), which are often separated by long periods of depression. Mood episodes may or may not also be accompanied by psychotic symptoms (delusions, hallucinations, thought disorder). It is subdivided into two types, bipolar I disorder, which involves manic episodes, and bipolar II disorder, which involves hypomanic episodes, which are periods of elevated mood less intense than full manic episodes.

Cathinone Molecule that closely resembles the amphetamine molecule (cathinone's other chemical name is beta-keto-amphetamine), and is found in nature most abundantly in the leaves of a plant called *khat* or *qat* (*Catha edulis*)

Central nervous system (CNS) depressants Any of the drugs that slow down the rate of neural transmission in the brain

Chronic disease Type of disease that cannot be cured but will continue to exist for the rest of the lifespan to a certain degree and therefore must be managed on a long-term basis

Chronic pain Pain that lasts longer than three to six months

Clinical trial Experiments or studies using new treatments on human subjects in order to establish scientific proof that 1) the new treatments actually work (efficacy), and 2) the new treatments are safe for human consumption

Coca **leaves** Leaves from any one of four different coca plants belonging to a family of plant species called the *erythroxylaceae*, chewed for millennia by indigenous peoples of South America for their ability to fight fatigue and suppress the appetite

Cocaine Naturally occurring stimulant molecule derived from coca leaves

Cognition Mental functions of the brain such as attention, decision making, planning, sensory perception, or calculation

Compulsion A strong urge to perform an action, even despite a conscious desire to not perform this action

Compulsivity Tendency to act in a manner that temporarily satisfies and removes deep urges or cravings

Conditioned stimulus In classical conditioning, a conditioned stimulus is produced by causing a neutral stimulus (such as a bell ringing) to occur at the same time and place as the unconditioned stimulus (food is brought out). The unconditioned stimulus produces a target behavior (salivation), and the subject (e.g., dog) thereby learns to associate the neutral stimulus with the unconditioned stimulus. Once this association is learned, the neutral stimulus is no longer neutral and thus becomes a conditioned stimulus.

Conditioning Processes by which new behaviors and new associations are learned

Controlled substance Legal terminology for the substances that the government has designated to have abuse potential and that require controlled and monitored distribution in order to prevent this abuse; includes both medications with potential for abuse as well as substances of abuse otherwise deemed to have no medical value

Controlled Substances Act (CSA) CSA is the shorthand term for the Comprehensive Drug Abuse Prevention and Control Act of 1970.

Counterfeit prescription drugs Illicit street drugs made with illegal pill presses to look like brand-name prescription drugs, sold on the black market

Craving A strong, continuous urge to partake of a food, beverage, or drug

Detoxification Method of slowly weaning a patient off a substance on which they have developed physical dependence either by slowly tapering off from that substance (e.g., slowly tapering off a benzodiazepine) or by administering and tapering off from a similar substance to which the patient has cross tolerance (e.g., administering a benzodiazepine to a patient with alcohol dependence to prevent withdrawal, and then slowly tapering off the benzodiazepine)

Detoxification The process of allowing a drug to leave the body system in order to end physical dependence on it

Diversion The illegal transfer of a legally obtained prescription drug from a patient to another person who uses it in an illicit way

Double-blind placebo-controlled studies The gold standard for establishing clinical effects of a medication, a type of randomized controlled trial in which a patient being treated for a certain condition (and who has signed up to participate in the research study) is randomly assigned by a researcher to receive a new drug being studied or a placebo. Neither the patient nor the clinician monitoring the patient's response to the drug is allowed to know if the patient has the drug or the placebo. This eliminates potential bias in the study.

Drug Any chemical substance that causes a change in the function of the body but is not food

Drug abuse Also known as **drug misuse**, this is the use of drugs in a way that is dangerous to oneself or to others; generally refers to psychoactive drugs that cause intoxication and/or may lead to addiction; can also refer to non-psychoactive performance-enhancing drugs such as androgenic-anabolic steroids

Drug class A set of drugs or medications with similar properties such as similar effects, chemical structures, or mechanisms or action

Drug dependence State in which a person has developed long-standing physical or psychological changes as the result of protracted substance use

Drug schedules Classification system used by the Drug Enforcement Agency (DEA) to categorize substances with abuse potential. Drugs are assigned to one of five schedules according to perceived abuse potential and medical utility. Schedule I drugs are considered by the DEA to have the highest abuse potential, and schedule V drugs are considered to have the lowest abuse potential.

Likewise, Schedule I drugs are considered to have no medical utility at all, whereas the other schedules all contain drugs regularly prescribed by physicians.

Drug-induced mania see mania

Drug-induced psychosis see psychosis

Drug-priming Use of a drug after a period of abstinence quickly causes a heavy return in craving for the drug, thus increasing the likelihood of restarting regular use

Efficacy Measurement of how well a drug works in accomplishing its stated purpose. During the drug development process, every new drug must be tested in several clinical trials to prove its true efficacy.

Endorphins Naturally occurring opiate molecules produced in the body and that serve functions such as rewarding behaviors and giving pain relief

Endorphins Opioids produced by a person's own body and that are involved in the regulation of pain and mood

Epidemic The rapid spread of a disease among a large number of people within a population in a short amount of time

Euphoria Feeling of happiness and well-being produced by the body's reward circuitry in the brain in response to perceived good behaviors; many illicit substances can produce a feeling of euphoria by directly activating cells in the brain

False binary A logical fallacy in which a debate is framed around two different positions that are presented as though they are the opposite of each other, suggesting that only a choice of one option or the other exists, when in reality, the two choices may be one of many options that exist—for example, if the choices exist on a spectrum of intermediate possibilities

Final common pathway of reward The reward system in the brain that is the ultimate destination of all reward signals (e.g., it is the same whether the body is rewarding exercise or drug use)

GABA$_A$ receptors Receptors in the brain that serve as the targets of benzodiazepines and other drugs. When activated, they increase the release of the neurotransmitter gamma-aminobutyric acid (GABA).

Gamma-aminobutyric acid (GABA) A type of neurotransmitter that slows and calms the nervous system, including the brain

Generalized anxiety disorder Anxiety disorder in which a person has excessive worries and fears about catastrophe occurring in numerous domains in their life (school, work, family, finances, relationships, etc.), and such worries are of a degree and intensity that it affects the person's ability to function in life

Habit Patterns of behavior that are learned through repetition and are often performed unconsciously; for example, a smoker might develop a habit of smoking a cigarette every morning before breakfast, such that it becomes part of his morning routine

Harm reduction Philosophy of drug policy that even though drug use is not the best choice, steps should be taken to reduce negative consequences related to it

Hospice centers Treatment facilities for patients approaching the end of their life to focus on ensuring their comfort as death approaches

Hyperalgesia Phenomenon that can occur in long-term use of opioid medications for pain in which the pain felt after stopping the opioids is actually more painful than the original pain felt before starting the opioid

Hypnotic [drug] Class of drugs that are primarily used to aid sleep

Illicit drug Any controlled substance used in an illegal way

Impulsivity Tendency to act toward obtaining an immediate reward without thought of long-term consequences

Intoxication Time-limited effect of a psychoactive drug that causes an alteration in the brain's function and results in an altered state of consciousness, leading to altered, sometimes dangerous behaviors

Judgment Mental ability to draw accurate conclusions about the world

Maintenance therapy A system by which those who have developed a drug addiction can treat the addiction

Major depressive disorder Disorder in which a person experiences depressive mood symptoms to a degree that causes functional impairment in their life, such as affecting her ability to work or function in relationships. Symptoms are of a time duration and level of intensity far beyond the normal sadness that all people feel from time to time. Symptoms must include two weeks or more of feeling sad or unable to experience pleasure. This must occur over half of the days. Other common depressive symptoms include insomnia, hopelessness, low energy, decreased concentration, decreased appetite, weight loss, slowing of movements, and suicidal thoughts.

Maladaptive coping strategies Strategies a person uses to cope with life's stressors but that involve additional significant negative consequences and that are ultimately not effective for the person; strategies that are appropriate at one stage of life may sometimes become maladaptive if carried on into later stages of life

Mandatory sentencing Popular laws passed in the 1980s and 1990s intended to deter drug use by imposing increasingly harsh minimum sentences for drug possession, often extending prison stays by years

Mania State of highly elevated mood in which a person experiences symptoms such as increased energy, decreased need for sleep, grandiose ideas, fast speech, racing thoughts, and increased impulsive behaviors such as sex with multiple partners, spending sprees, drug use, or violent acts. Seen in bipolar I disorder and schizoaffective disorder, bipolar type.

Medication assisted therapy (MAT) Term for maintenance programs using prescription drugs to replace street drugs in the treatment of addictions, such as using methadone or buprenorphine to treat addiction to illegal opioids, thus allowing the user to escape time-consuming and often illegal activities they pursue in order to maintain their addictions

Medicine Legal drugs taken with the purpose of treating or preventing disease

Mental illness Any illness that causes a change in a person's thinking or behavior

Molecular signaling Process by which cells in the body use molecules to communicate with other cells in the body by activating receptors; essentially all medicines are molecules and work by using molecular signaling to change different processes in the body

Molecules Collections of atoms that bond together to form larger structures that each have their unique properties

Narcolepsy Neurological disorder where a person has periods of excessive sleepiness during the day due to a disruption in the sleep-wake cycle

Narcotic Imprecise term commonly used to mean any illegal street drug; currently, the Drug Enforcement Agency officially defines this term as synonymous with the word "opioid"

Needle exchange programs (NEPs) Also known as needle and syringe program (NSPs) or syringe exchange programs (SEPs), NEPs are programs that provide clean needles and syringes, alcohol swabs and pads, and sterile water to people who are already using injection drugs in order to help decrease the spread of infectious diseases such as HIV.

Nervous system Organ system in the body that contains nerve tissue and is comprised of a central nervous system, which includes the brain and spinal cord, and the peripheral nervous system, which includes sensory and motor neurons to the skin, muscles, and other tissues not in the central nervous system

Neurons Cells of the nervous system that can transmit electrical signals to other cells in the body; these cells are the principal functional components of the nervous system and make up organs such as the brain and spinal cord

Neutral stimulus A stimulus that does not cause a target behavior

Opiates Naturally occurring opioid molecules isolated from the opium poppy and used in medicine, for example, morphine or codeine

Opioid drugs Class of drugs whose members have similar properties and chemical structures to the naturally occurring opiate molecules, derived from the *papaver somniferum* plant. Includes both naturally occurring opiate molecules as well as synthetic and semisynthetic opioid molecules that have been synthesized using laboratory methods

Opioid receptors Receptors on cells in the body that respond to opioid medications and endorphins and cause changes in the body, such as decreasing pain, increasing sleepiness, decreasing the movement of the digestive tract, and more.

Opium alkaloids A group of similarly shaped molecules found in the opium poppy that are directly useful either as pharmaceuticals or as chemical precursors for other medicines

Opium poppy Flowering plant *papaver somniferum* that is the primary source of naturally occurring opioid molecules called opium alkaloids

Overdose The taking of a drug in a quantity larger than that which is safe, resulting in possible harmful and toxic effects, including death

Pain As per the International Association for the Study of Pain, it is defined as "an unpleasant sensory and emotional experience associated with actual or potential tissue damage, or described in terms of such damage"

Palliative care Branch of medicine that focuses on patient comfort for those who have incurable or terminal illnesses

Panic disorder Anxiety disorder in which a person gets "panic attacks" of overwhelming anxiety, accompanied by thoughts such that the person thinks she is dying or losing her mind

Patent medicines A large category of medications that were sold before the 1910s before the period were commercially sold; no prescription required, name-brand medicines produced before the era of drug regulation that did not have to disclose their ingredients

Patient satisfaction Model to measure quality of patient care that became popular in the United State in the 2000s in which surveys of patients' satisfaction with their care at a hospital are used to determine the quality of care at that institution and to determine the amount that payers would reimburse that institution. Often criticized for having little to do with actual good medical outcome.

Performance enhancers Drugs used to improve performance in specific activities, such as academics or athletics, as opposed to drugs used as medicines, which treat or prevent disease

Physical addiction Physical component of addiction that reinforces repeated use of a substance through mechanisms such as tolerance, physical dependence, and avoidance of withdrawal

Physical dependence State in which a person has developed physical tolerance to a substance and where continued use of it is required to avoid a withdrawal syndrome

Pill mill Term for clinics presenting themselves as pain-management centers but in reality function as money-making operations that give out prescriptions for controlled substances without requiring a proper medical reason

Polysubstance use The use of more than one psychoactive substance at the same time

Prefrontal cortex The area of the brain closest the forehead where many of the brain's "executive functions" are performed—that is, where mental functions such as organizing, planning, and attention are primarily located

Prescription drugs Drugs that in general are legally obtained only through receiving a prescription by a practitioner such as a medical doctor and then by getting the prescription filled at a pharmacy

Property crimes Include burglary, larceny, motor vehicle theft, and arson, and increase as a result of increased drug use

Psychoactive drugs Drugs that affect the function of the brain that results in altered states of consciousness, changes in perception, mood, and behavior

Psychological addiction Psychological component of addiction that reinforces repeated use of a substance through mechanisms such as habits, environmental triggers, impulsivity-compulsivity, etc.

Psychological dependence Involves the presence of 1) learned behaviors that can be set off by numerous environmental triggers in a person's life and environment that will cause him or her to want to take a drug, and 2) an altered baseline mood and sense of well-being.

Psychosis State of consciousness in which a person experiences symptoms such as delusions, hallucinations, and thought disorder. Thought disorder results in disorganized speech, such that the person's thoughts do not follow a logical or linear progression, and sentences and words spoken may consist of completely unrelated topics. Can be caused by mental illness, medical illness, or be drug-induced.

Public health The approach to health that analyzes health at a population level in order to prevent disease and promote wellness through coordination of activities in communities, organizations, governments, and societies

Raw opium Product made from the opium poppy since ancient times in which the sap, or "latex," of the flower bud is dried and collected

Receptors Structures found in cells that cause changes in the cell in response to molecular signals

Recreational drug Any drug used for pleasurable effects, as opposed to drugs used as medicines, which treat or prevent disease

Recreational use The use of drugs for pleasurable effects, as opposed to medical drug use such as treating or preventing disease

Relapse The reactivation of an addiction after a period of abstinence or remission

Remission Stage of a chronic disease in which no more symptoms remain, but preventive measures must still be taken to prevent relapse

Rewarding behavior Behavior that the brain interprets as positive and produces an enjoyable feeling, which reinforces the person to perform that behavior again to obtain the reward again

Schizoaffective disorder Disorder in which a person has periods of psychotic symptoms (delusions, hallucinations, thought disorder) as well as periods of mood disturbance (mania or depression). To distinguish from bipolar disorder or major depressive disorder, the person must have periods of psychosis in which no mood symptoms are present at the same time. Subdivided into schizoaffective disorder, bipolar type; and schizoaffective disorder, depressive type.

Schizophrenia Disorder in which a person develops chronic psychosis (delusions, hallucinations, thought disorder); begins in early adulthood and generally progressively worsens throughout the lifespan

Scofflaw A word coined during the Prohibition era to describe an irreverent attitude toward the government in which the general authority of the law was respected less

Sedative [drug] see **sedative-hypnotics**

Sedative-hypnotics Drug class whose overall effects are *relaxing* (sedative) and *sleep-inducing* (hypnotic); also known as anxiolytics, sedatives, or tranquillizers for their ability to relieve nervousness and make a person feel tranquil

Self-medication Hypothesis of addiction that people begin using substances of abuse as a form of self-treatment for physical pain or mental anguish. In the long run, users may find the strategy was maladaptive since they find themselves facing unintended consequences; the use of illicit or street drugs by a person in an attempt to cope with a legitimate physical or mental health concern

Semisynthetic opioids Novel opioid molecules not found in nature and created by chemists by taking naturally occurring opium alkaloids and using chemical reactions to slightly alter their shapes

Set and setting The mindset and physical setting of a person during use of a drug

Specific phobia A strong and excessive fear of a specific object or situation, such as fear of flying so strong as to make the person completely unable to board a plane

Stigma Strong societal disapproval or disdain for a particular group of people

Stimulants Drugs that increase the level of arousal in the nervous system and produce effects such as increased value medically and nonmedically for their ability to increase wakefulness, focus, concentration, and motivation

Street drugs Substances of abuse illegally sold by drug dealers through the black market and that have not been subjected to safety guarantees

Substance use disorder Diagnosis indicating a patient has a potentially dangerous pattern of substance intoxication or has an addiction to a substance

Sympathetic nervous system Portion of the nervous system that becomes activated in response to danger, resulting in physiologic changes to prepare the person for "fight or flight"

Synthetic opioids Novel opioid molecules that were synthesized in laboratories from non-opiate molecules but that nonetheless can activate opioid receptors

Tolerance Occurs when the body requires ever-increasing amounts of a drug in order to achieve the same effect

Tranquilizers see **sedative-hypnotics**

Twin studies Studies looking at health outcomes of identical twins who had been adopted into separate foster homes; hence, studies comparing people with identical genomes but raised in different environments

Unconditioned stimulus In classical conditioning, a naturally occurring stimulus that reliably produces a target behavior in the subject

Violent crime Any crime that involves the use of violent force or the threat of such violence on a victim. Includes murder, rape, physical assault, armed robbery, kidnapping, and others.

Withdrawal A physiologic process that occurs as a result of quickly stopping use of a drug in a person who had developed physical dependence

Withdrawal syndrome Specific set of symptoms produced during withdrawal of a specific drug; the symptoms in the withdrawal syndrome are generally the opposite of the types of effects the person felt when taking the drugs

Z-drugs Drug class of mostly sleep-inducing drugs similar to benzodiazepines

Sources for Further Information

The following is a short list of resources useful for further information on topics presented in this text.

Addiction Treatment Resources

The Substance Abuse and Mental Health Services Administration (SAMHSA) website is an excellent resource to search for addiction treatment resources available in one's geographical area. The website also provides access to the large amounts of substance use data collected by the organization annually. https://www.samhsa.gov/

Narcotics Anonymous (NA) a traditional, group-based, 12-step model of addiction treatment. Members support each other in their cessation efforts. Sessions are free and are found all across the world. www.na.org

General Information on Substance Abuse

The National Survey on Drug Use and Health (NSDUH) is given annually to collect information and statistics about the nation's current substance use. The data from these surveys are compiled into a highly detailed report that allows for an intricate and specific view of current drug abuse. These data are frequently utilized and cited by addiction researchers and policy makers. https://www.samhsa.gov/data/data-we-collect/nsduh-national-survey-drug-use-and-health

Drug Abuse Warning Network (DAWN) is another important method by which SAMHSA collects data about substance use. DAWN collects data about all drug-related hospital emergency department visits. This serves as a type of approximate measure for the amount of harm that drugs are causing each year. https://www.samhsa.gov/data/data-we-collect/dawn-drug-abuse-warning-network

United States Department of Justice National Drug Threat Assessment (NDTA) is a document created each year by the DEA to monitor illicit drug abuse and to assess the dangers these drugs pose to the general population. It describes the origins of illicit drugs, such as which criminal organizations produce and distribute each type of illicit drug.
www.dea.gov

Dreamland. This nonfiction work by journalist Sam Quinones offers a more in-depth examination of the origins and the ravages of the opioid crisis. It explores the roles played by pharmaceutical companies, drug cartels, individual drug users, and more. At the same time, it succeeds at bringing a more human face to the opioid crisis thanks to numerous interviews and stories by the people most directly involved.
Quinones, Sam. *Dreamland: The True Tale of America's Opiate Epidemic.* New York: Bloomsbury Press, 2015.

The Addiction Solution: Treating Our Dependence on Opioids and Other Drugs is a book recently published by Dr. Lloyd Sederer, an addiction psychiatrist at Columbia University in New York City and one of the leaders in the field of addiction. This book calls for a cultural shift in the way society deals with addiction and offers numerous practical and progressive ideas to reform policy toward substances with abuse potential.

Sederer, Lloyd I., *The Addiction Solution: Treating Our Dependence on Opioids and Other Drugs.* New York: Scribner, 2018.

Index

ABOUT THE AUTHORS

Robert L. Bryant, MD, is a PGY3 psychiatry resident at Montefiore Medical Center/Albert Einstein College of Medicine in the Bronx, New York.

Howard L. Forman, MD, directs the Addiction Consultation Service at Montefiore Medical Center and is assistant professor of psychiatry at Albert Einstein College of Medicine in the Bronx, New York. Board certified in psychiatry, forensic psychiatry, and addiction medicine.